T0383693

"*Understanding and Coping with Illness Anxiety* is an essential guide that normalizes and beautifully articulates this commonly misunderstood yet widely experienced problem. Phil Lane provides an accessible, reader friendly exploration of illness anxiety, with practical and relatable information. Highly recommended to anyone seeking to gain a deeper understanding of themselves and find relief."

Melissa Collins, LCSW, LCADC, *Psychotherapist*

"Phil Lane has written an important addition to the available resources on anxiety. This book will be of great help to patients and practitioners alike."

Charles Bachus, PhD, *Clinical Psychologist*

Understanding and Coping with Illness Anxiety

This book is both a clinical and accessible guide, offering comfort and psychoeducation to readers as well as needed psychological explanation of concepts to mental health and medical professionals.

In the continually evolving aftermath of the global pandemic, the importance of understanding how disease, illness, and health affect our emotional and mental well-being, and how each influences the other, cannot be overstated. The book is divided into four sections: (1) an accessible yet detailed description of what illness anxiety is and its diagnostic criteria, including case examples; (2) a practically applicable description and delineation of coping strategies for managing illness-related anxiety, including bullet points and diagrams; (3) a section describing how patients heal from illness anxiety disorder, including case examples; and (4) a section containing practical exercises, meditations, and activities to assist the reader in learning coping strategies. This section can also be utilized by mental health professionals to use for treatment with their clients. This book is a relevant, timely, and needed resource that will highlight an underrepresented area of the psychological literature.

Phil Lane, MSW, LCSW, is a licensed clinical social worker and psychotherapist in private practice. He specializes in treating anxiety, depression, and mood disorders. He lives and practices in Central New Jersey.

Routledge Focus on Mental Health

Routledge Focus on Mental Health presents short books on current topics, linking in with cutting-edge research and practice.

For a full list of titles in this series, please visit www.routledge.com/Routle dge-Focus-on-Mental-Health/book-series/RFMH

Titles in the series:

Understanding and Coping with Illness Anxiety

Phil Lane

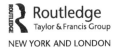

Routledge
Taylor & Francis Group

NEW YORK AND LONDON

First published 2024
by Routledge
605 Third Avenue, New York, NY 10158

and by Routledge
4 Park Square, Milton Park, Abingdon, Oxon, OX14 4RN

Routledge is an imprint of the Taylor & Francis Group, an informa business

ISBN: 9781032637914 (hbk)
ISBN: 9781032683966 (pbk)
ISBN: 9781032637921 (ebk)

DOI: 10.4324/9781032637921

Typeset in Times New Roman
by Newgen Publishing UK

Dedicated in loving memory to Carmela (Sandy), Joseph, and Matthew

Disclaimer

The case examples provided in this book are based on the experiences of real patients, whose names and identities have been changed to protect their privacy. Any resemblance to actual persons is entirely coincidental. The information provided in this book is for informational purposes only and is not intended to replace medical diagnosis or treatment.

Author Biography

Phil Lane is a licensed clinical social worker and psychotherapist in private practice. He holds a bachelor's degree in English and a master's degree in social work. Phil specializes in the treatment of anxiety, panic, depression, and mood disorders. As a humanistic and existential psychotherapist, Phil practices with an emphasis on empathy and compassion. Phil and his wife live in Central New Jersey.

Contents

Preface

"I feel messed up." That was the only way I could think to describe it when the doctor asked why I was there, why I had pleaded with the office for a same-day appointment, why I was back so soon after my last visit. When he asked me to be more specific, I pointed out a few particular symptoms I was experiencing: "I feel dizzy, wobbly, short of breath, it's hard to swallow. I just feel … off." The doctor poked and prodded a bit, checked this and that, but ultimately told me I seemed fine. He added that I was young, seemed healthy, and should not worry. I left the appointment with no answers and little belief that I was, actually, fine.

A few weeks later, I spent a night in the emergency room, complaining of the same vague symptoms. Tests were ordered. I was wheeled here and there for X-rays and scans, specialists came and went. I was discharged the next day with a clean bill of health and a sizeable bill for services.

This did not assuage my fears that I had a serious medical problem. At the time, I did not realize that what I was experiencing was not a physical problem but, rather, a physical response to intense emotions. I was constantly stressed, tired, worried, angry, and uncertain—and my body could tell, so it reacted. It tried to warn me and keep me safe. The problem was that the signals were crossed: my body was responding to an imagined danger.

I am relieved to report that more than a decade since this experience, I no longer persistently worry that I am afflicted with some horrific, incurable medical condition. Don't get me wrong—I still get anxious, tired, worried, angry, and unsure at times. But it doesn't overwhelm me like it once did. And my body doesn't overreact the way it used to. This book is for anyone who has been frightened by physical symptoms, overwhelmed by their body's response to anxiety, or convinced that they are suffering a serious medical problem. There is hope. There is soothing and healing. There is a way to feel safe again.

—Phil Lane

Now, there is no one who does not know that the ideas … of pain, which are formed in our thought when bodies from without touch us, bear no resemblance whatever to those bodies.

—René Descartes

Acknowledgments

I wish to thank the following people, all of whom played an important role in the writing of this book: Nicole Lane, for her unwavering support, reassurance, cheerleading, and tireless patience. Amanda Savage, editor at Routledge Publishing, for her guidance and insight and for championing this book. Daniel Beck for his assistance and knowledge throughout the post-writing process. Jacqueline Parkison for her editorial eye and acute attention to detail. Professors Jacki Szabo, Dr. John McTighe, and Joann McEniry for their support and advocacy of this project. The numerous therapists who have helped me over the years with learning how to manage anxiety and who have served as professional mentors. Thank you, also, to all of my clients—past and present—from whom I continue to learn and grow as a clinician.

Acronyms and Abbreviations

CBT	Cognitive behavioral therapy
CDC	Centers for Disease Control and Prevention
DBT	Dialectical behavioral therapy
DSM-5-TR	Diagnostic and Statistical Manual of Mental Disorders, Fifth Edition, Text Revision
HIPPA	Health Insurance Portability and Accountability Act
IAD	Illness anxiety disorder
IBS	Irritable bowel syndrome
LAC	Licensed associate counselor
LCSW	Licensed clinical social worker
LMFT	Licensed marriage and family therapist
LMHC	Licensed mental health counselor
LPC	Licensed professional counselor
MBCT	Mindfulness-based cognitive therapy
PMHNP	Psychiatric-mental health nurse practitioner
PsyD	Clinical psychologist
REBT	Rational-emotive behavioral therapy

1 Understanding Illness Anxiety Disorder

Defining Illness Anxiety

Colin, a 20-year-old college student, started therapy after having dropped out of school in the middle of his junior year. He was, by all accounts, a strong student with a healthy social life; he achieved good grades and adjusted well to being away from home. The prior spring, he had experienced a fainting spell while in an airport preparing to fly home for break. He was rushed to the hospital by ambulance and underwent a battery of tests. Though he was subsequently cleared by doctors, a nagging, persistent fear remained with him. Colin's sense of safety regarding his physical health had been shattered.

Colin is representative of many individuals who struggle with illness anxiety. So common is the problem that in the latest iteration of the Diagnostic and Statistical Manual of Mental Disorders, Fifth Edition, Text Revision (DSM-5-TR), it has a clinically accepted name: illness anxiety disorder (IAD).[1] This is a well-deserved update from what was once known as "hypochondriasis" or "neurosis." No longer do we view this as a problem afflicting "neurotic," "histrionic," or "attention-seeking" people; rather, we see it as a subset of anxiety with a particular and narrow focus on one's physical health and a persistent fear of acquiring a serious illness.

Anxiety, in a generalized sense, is a fear of "what if." From a cognitive behavioral therapy perspective, to the anxious person, the fear that it *could* happen is as real as if it *is* happening.[2] In the case of IAD, "I *feel* like I'm dying" can quickly and easily become "I *am* dying." In a nutshell, this is how anxiety works: it ignores the present and often obscures the facts that might keep an individual feeling safe and secure. For Colin, no amount of medical tests or clinical reassurance could convince him that he was safe. Once he had experienced the frightening event in the airport, he simply could not believe that something catastrophic was not waiting in the wings.

What is it about our personal health that creates such fertile ground for anxious thinking? Perhaps it is that we are in our bodies all day and for all of our lives; we rely on our bodies to function without incident at every level,

DOI: 10.4324/9781032637921-1

from molecular to cellular and so on. When they struggle to function or when a system encounters a problem, it can feel jarring, frightening, and uncertain. Anxiety thrives in such conditions. There is, however, a larger fear that underlies our health anxiety: a fear of nonexistence. Nearly a century ago, Sigmund Freud posited that one of the base human fears is the fear of physiological decay, illness, and death.[3] This human fear has not changed, but the ease of inundating ourselves with reminders of its lurking presence has multiplied exponentially. We live in a culture that has monetized and commercialized "well-being" and "health" to such an extent that concern for our physical health has grown into an often unmanageable worry. We seek answers, diagnoses, and treatments from questionable sources, such as the omnipresent "Dr. Google." We stress and fret about our health, which ironically has a negative impact on the very part of ourselves that we are trying so diligently to protect.

DSM-5-TR Criteria for Illness Anxiety Disorder

- Preoccupation with having or acquiring a serious illness.
- Somatic symptoms are not present or, if present, are only mild in intensity. If another medical condition is present or there is a high risk for developing a medical condition (e.g., strong family history is present), the preoccupation is clearly excessive or disproportionate.
- There is a high level of anxiety about health, and the individual is easily alarmed about personal health status.
- The individual performs excessive health-related behaviors (e.g., repeatedly checks his or her body for signs of illness) or exhibits maladaptive avoidance (e.g., avoids doctor appointments and hospitals).
- Illness preoccupation has been present for at least six months, but the specific illness that is feared may change over that period of time.
- The illness-related preoccupation is not better explained by another mental disorder, such as somatic symptom disorder, panic disorder, generalized anxiety disorder, body dysmorphic disorder, obsessive-compulsive disorder, or delusional disorder, somatic type.

Specify whether:
- Care-seeking type: Medical care, including physician visits or undergoing tests and procedures, is frequently used.
- Care-avoidant type: Medical care is rarely used.

Reprinted with permission from the Diagnostic and Statistical Manual of Mental Disorders, fifth edition, DSM-V, p. 315 (Copyright © 2013). American Psychiatric Association. All Rights Reserved.

Colin met many of the DSM-5-TR criteria for a clinical diagnosis of IAD. He was disproportionately preoccupied with having or acquiring a serious illness; he was easily alarmed about his personal health status; he routinely performed health-related behaviors such as checking his body for changes, abnormalities, or signs of illness.

Care-Seeking vs. Care-Avoidant IAD

For Colin and others who struggle with illness anxiety, the resultant anxiety-based behaviors are often directed to one extreme or the other: constant answer-seeking or a resigned acceptance of a medical "fact" that it is actually a drastic and incorrect conclusion drawn from anxiety.

The subtype of Colin's diagnosis was "care-seeking type," meaning he frequently utilized doctor's visits and medical testing to seek reassurance. The other extreme is termed "care-avoidant type." Both are anxiety-driven responses, as one is an overutilization of medical care and the other, an underutilization.

Care-Seeking IAD

The cost of care-seeking IAD can be high, both monetarily and emotionally. Some individuals will spend thousands of dollars on medical bills, out-of-pocket payments, and unnecessary tests. Those who visit emergency rooms are often left with exorbitant bills for short and often inconclusive stays, and hospitals, particularly emergency departments, can be relentless about receiving payment. A 2016 study shares a case of a Saudi man who spent more than $175,000 undergoing unneeded medical tests and scans due to an unfounded fear of having cancer.[4]

The emotional price of care-seeking can be equally high. As an individual receives more care yet fewer answers, they may slowly become depressed and hopeless, distrustful of doctors and the medical profession. When the people and places they go to for answers consistently turn them away with no conclusions, they, understandably, become jaded. This can quickly escalate to a feeling of isolation and bring about further maladaptive responses such as expanding the geographical area of their search for diagnostic answers, locating medical offices and urgent care centers that do not accept insurance and require out-of-pocket payments, seeking answers from unreliable sources such as the Internet, and self-diagnosing. The cumulative impact of these behaviors can be a growing sense of hopelessness and a persistent, unmanageable feeling of catastrophic worry. People with the care-seeking subtype of IAD will often:

- Visit numerous doctor's offices for medical opinions and diagnoses
- Visit hospital emergency departments or urgent care centers when primary care appointments are not immediately available

- Seek second opinions from multiple medical professionals
- Engage in constant Internet research on symptoms and diagnoses

Certain types of medical specialists are often overutilized by care-seeking patients. These include the following specialists.

Cardiologists

Because anxiety is often felt in the heart and chest, some anxious patients seek out cardiologists out of fear that they are having a heart attack or other heart-related medical problem.

Neurologists

When an anxious patient experiences frightening symptoms in their head, they may turn to neurology specialists out of fear that they have a tumor or other serious neurological problem.

Gastroenterologists

Anxiety commonly manifests in the stomach and digestive systems, so patients may undergo unnecessary testing of their GI systems to explore a feared intestinal or digestive problem.

Care-Avoidant IAD

Individuals with care-avoidant IAD live in a resigned state akin to that of someone with a terminal illness. They have accepted what they believe to be their fate; the problem, however, is that this fate is a creation of their anxious mind. The emotional cost is often the overwhelming sense of resignation: a letting-go of the importance previously given to areas of life such as career, social connection, and daily sense of purpose, which becomes a narrowing of their sphere of existence. It also leaves the patient completely alone with their anxious thoughts and assumptions. It also leaves the patient susceptible to depression and heightened anxiety as they wait for the "inevitable" to occur. People with the care-avoidant subtype of IAD will often:

- Avoid doctor's visits and medical appointments
- Develop a complete aversion to medical or health information, even that which might be necessary or helpful

Both care-seeking and care-avoidant patients must work toward a renewed feeling of safety and security regarding their physical health (Figure 1.1).

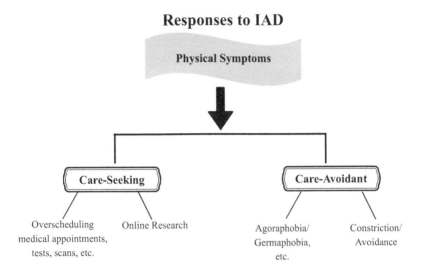

Figure 1.1 Flow chart illustrating the two main responses to illness anxiety, care-seeking, and care-avoidance.

Differential Diagnosis

IAD is not and should not be treated as a disorder of manipulation, narcissism, or attention-seeking, though it can often be misinterpreted as such. The person with IAD is severely anxious, not narcissistic, delusional, or self-centered. There are, however, two similar diagnoses that may be conflated with IAD: factitious disorder and somatic symptom disorder.

The psychological root of factitious disorder is deception, wherein the individual uses a false diagnosis to misrepresent themself, often for an external reward. This may be done to elicit sympathy or for a financial or material benefit. Therapists who misdiagnose IAD as factitious disorder run the serious risk of mislabeling and pathologizing patients and, therefore, tainting the therapeutic process. Factitious disorder imposed on another (previously "factitious disorder by proxy") involves the patient assigning physical or psychological symptoms onto others (often children, family members, or pets), in, again, an effort to be deceptive. Factitious disorder involves falsifying symptoms, whereas IAD is more akin to overanalysis and misinterpretation (and, therefore, misrepresentation) of symptoms without the intent of deceit.

Somatic symptom disorder describes a response to symptoms such as actual physical pain with an overanalysis of their meaning. This differentiates from IAD in that there often is an actual, not imagined physical symptom. In IAD, there is either no symptom or an extremely mild symptom that to the non-anxious mind would cause little to no concern. Mental health professionals must be careful not to confuse these similar diagnoses or to rush to one before receiving and understanding the full and appropriate information about the patient.

Whom Illness Anxiety Affects

Anxiety related to physical health and fear of illness does not discriminate. We are susceptible to illness from the moment we are born, maybe even before that. It is a constant possibility to become ill, and therefore, for some, it becomes a constant worry. Self-protection can be traced back to a primitive level and is an innate human response to dangerous or frightening stimuli. Early humans fought, fled, and sheltered when they were threatened, and those primitive responses remain with us, even in our comparatively advanced state. In current psychological parlance, we describe these responses as "fight, flight, and freeze."

In our current time, we are no longer at daily risk of attack by wild predators, but these dangers have been replaced by others. Disease and illness provoke similar primitive responses within us when we feel threatened by them. Some who fear illness move directly toward it in the form of care-seeking (we might consider this a fight response). Others directly avoid care when faced with the potentiality of illness (we may view this as a flight response). Still others resign themselves to their fate, taking no action whatsoever (we might term this a freeze response). All three of these responses pose risks as they are either overreactions or underreactions to the situation. Taken to extremes, they become unhealthy, or maladaptive, and can directly lead to disordered thinking and cognitive patterns and, if persistent and disruptive, to IAD.

While all humans share a tendency toward each or all of the primitive fear responses at some point, only some respond in such an extreme fashion that it results in a diagnosable psychological disorder. Anxiety disorders in particular affect a wide swath of the population. Given our society's constant sense of unrest and uncertainty, it is no surprise that many people's lives are disrupted by persistent anxiety and worry. The COVID-19 pandemic reaffirmed and highlighted the notion that illness and fear of illness acquisition can be one of the major causes of anxiety and its associated disorders.

Specific At-Risk Populations

Children

Early experiences often formulate and influence later anxieties and aversions. A child's early medical experiences are formative in how they view medical treatment later in life. For instance, a child who has a negative experience receiving an injection may form a lifelong aversion to doctor's visits or to needles. Additionally, how a child is parented leaves an imprint on their ability to feel safe with their physical health. If, for example, a child's parent is dismissive or invalidating of their feelings when they experience physical pain or injury, they may grow up to feel unsafe and uncertain regarding their health and, therefore, become care-seeking or care-avoidant.

Adolescents/Young Adults

Teens and emerging adults are highly susceptible to media influence, which can result in a tendency to self-diagnose both psychological and medical problems. Self-diagnosis can lead to misinterpretation and incorrect conclusions about symptoms and cause incongruent fear and anxiety about one's health status. While social media platforms such as Reddit and TikTok can help young people feel commonality and connection, they can also be sources of misinformation, particularly regarding mental and physical health symptoms. A 2022 *New York Times* article supports this idea:

> In recent years, discussions about mental health have proliferated on social media, particularly on TikTok, where the format allows for easily digestible, intimate videos that appear in a never-ending algorithmic feed. And for those researching various disorders, it has become increasingly easy to find bite-sized definitions and self-assessment quizzes online. While this bounty of unfiltered resources can serve to reduce the stigma associated with mental illness, there are downsides.[5]

The LGBTQIA2+ and BIPOC Communities

Feeling shamed and judged, unfortunately, can cause some individuals to avoid medical treatment. All individuals, regardless of sexual orientation, race, ethnicity, or lifestyle, deserve to be treated with empathy, compassion, and understanding. Some patients from these communities report feeling "othered" by the medical profession, meaning that the provider "makes a rigid distinction between the provider's and the patient's community."[6] People who feel shamed, "othered," or marginalized by the medical profession may develop skepticism and, therefore, become anxious or avoidant about seeking necessary medical treatment.

Laborers/Athletes/Other Professionals

Those individuals who use their bodies daily as a part of their livelihood understandably can become overly protective of their health. While a certain level of attention is, of course, healthy, this can, when taken to an extreme, result in an obsessive and unhealthy attention to one's physical health as well as an overreliance on exercise or preventative care. Understanding an individual's career and its impact on their emotional health is an important aspect of treatment, as it can help us understand why some individuals may be more prone to health-related anxiety based upon their career circumstances.

Seniors

There is a level of normalcy to fear related to aging and death, but taken to an emotional extreme, this fear can cause avoidance of necessary medical checkups and follow-ups. For the geriatric population, the medical profession's understanding of the feelings of vulnerability around aging is important in ensuring that these individuals do not become frightened or avoidant of medical treatment.

Traumatic and Epigenetic Causes of Illness Anxiety

Why does a person with obsessive-compulsive disorder check and recheck that the stove is off? The simple answer is that they are worried and, therefore, hypervigilant or "on guard." Imagine a smoke detector that is so sensitive it goes off if you simply strike a match or blow out a candle. Such is the case with anxiety; it trains us to be on the lookout at all times for every possible contingency or eventuality. It reacts with hair-trigger urgency, responding to every stimulus, no matter how minor. When it comes to our physical health, small changes such as unexpected aches and pains or unexplained skin changes such as rashes or bumps can convince us of a larger, potentially catastrophic problem.

But why are some individuals able to "roll with" and not overreact to physical symptoms and changes while others are sucked into a vortex of worry and catastrophic thinking? We might view the answer through two separate yet related lenses: *trauma* (disturbing events that negatively influence our thoughts, attitudes, behaviors, and other aspects of functioning) and *epigenetics* (environmental and psychosocial factors, such as early childhood experiences or exposure to toxins, that interact with physiology). Both, in a general sense, explain the ways in which outer events and circumstances affect our inner lives and formulate our healthy or unhealthy responses to stimuli.

Trauma

When he was in his early 30s, Jason witnessed a colleague suffer a fatal heart attack. For Jason, this event created a pervasive and persistent feeling that anything could happen to anyone at any time. It was not long after witnessing the event that Jason began to experience tightness in his chest and heart palpitations. Though he knew rationally that he was most likely not suffering a heart attack as his coworker had, Jason's anxious mind would often convince him otherwise. Jason underwent medical testing, sought constant professional advice, and found himself never completely convinced that something was not physically wrong with him.

In her seminal book *Trauma and Recovery*, Dr. Judith Herman writes of three distinct stages that occur following a traumatic event: hypervigilance, constriction, and numbing.[7] All three commonly occur in IAD individuals. For Jason, hypervigilance was an immediate response to the traumatic stimulus. He became hyperaware of protecting himself against further disaster through the overutilization of medical advice-seeking and the constant checking of symptoms and bodily sensations. Jason also constricted, or narrowed, his life; his constant, obsessive attention to physical symptoms detracted from his ability to be present in other areas of his life. He would also numb himself through distraction, working long hours as a way to be engaged in something other than his feelings of worry and dread. Herman writes that the goal of trauma recovery is returning to a sense of safety and a reconnection with everyday life. Jason was ultimately able to do so, but not before experiencing the life-disrupting aftereffects of the traumatic event.

Epigenetics

Epigenetic influences do not alter an individual's genetic code; rather, they affect an individual's psychological development and later functioning. This noncoding DNA has been proven to be affected by environmental stressors, which can include stressful emotions.[8] Take, for instance, two identical twins; while they share the same genetics and genomes, their unique life experiences will formulate how they adapt to, cope with, and manage life situations. While these unique life experiences may include traumatic events and inherited or generational trauma, it is the confluence of genetics, events, and environment that epigenetically shapes an individual.

When Michelle, now middle-aged, was a child, her mother battled, and ultimately succumbed to, lung cancer. She was surrounded by her mother's illness for many of the formative years of her life. She had witnessed up close her mother's slow, painful journey through chemotherapy, radiation, hospice care, and death at the young age of 55. Having spent many years in an environment whose central theme was illness, Michelle became deeply affected and frightened by the potentiality of becoming terminally ill herself.

For Jason, one specific, traumatic *event* activated IAD; for Michelle, an *environment* of illness and disease was the activating force. Samantha, whose situation will be further explained in the following section, is another example of the epigenetic influence. As a heavily industrialized and polluted area, Samantha's environment had a significant impact on her health-related fears. The daily sights of smokestacks and factories imprinted Samantha with a sense of doom regarding her physical well-being, and this surrounding environment exacerbated her illness-related anxiety. Epigenetics, in a psychological sense, has to do with our unique life experiences and how they formulate and affect our functioning.

Other Contributors to IAD

While trauma and epigenetics are common contributory factors, there are a number of other contributors to the development of illness-related anxiety.

Chronic Pain

Some people suffer with constant, daily chronic pain yet are, overall, healthy. However, persistent pain can trick us into concluding that something deeper and more serious is occurring in our body. Many who experience chronic pain spend a great deal of time, energy, and money trying to find the origin of the symptoms, to no avail. Symptoms of chronic pain such as backaches or joint pain can easily be misinterpreted as more serious problems. When the focus shifts from trying to *find* the cause of the pain to learning to *manage* the pain, the patient often feels relief and lessened anxiety.

Autoimmune Disorders

Certain autoimmune disorders have been scientifically shown to contribute to psychological problems such as depression and anxiety. A 2021 study in *The Mediterranean Journal of Rheumatology* found that neuropsychiatric problems such as depression and anxiety were prevalent in between 21% and 95% of patients with the autoimmune disorder systemic lupus erythematosus.[9] These disorders, much like chronic pain, are long-lasting and persistent, so resignation, exhaustion, depression, and anxiety are commonly experienced by patients, as well as a fear of the condition worsening or leading to more serious complications. Further, those with autoimmune disorders are more susceptible to a wide range of illnesses and, therefore, more susceptible to illness-related anxiety.

Attachment/Parenting

The consistency or inconsistency of how we were parented plays a significant role in how we manage and cope with anxiety and fear. If, for instance, a parent is inconsistent in their presence or in their style of disciplining or caregiving, a child may respond with an "anxious" attachment style, meaning that they will often feel uncertain of whether they will receive comfort or rebuke in a time of need. A child who sometimes receives comfort when upset and other times receives punishment will be unsure of which to expect and, therefore, anxious.

Connected to IAD, this can affect a person's ability to feel safe or comforted when anxious or frightened. This, then, can lead to care-seeking behaviors, as an individual may desperately seek reassurance from an "authority" figure such as a doctor or medical professional.

Scrupulosity/Moralistic OCD

For some anxious patients, an illness or disease being visited upon them can be interpreted as a form of "paying the piper" or "atoning for their sins." Michelle, the woman mentioned prior, was a former cigarette smoker like her mother, and she would sometimes convince herself that death from lung cancer was to be her fate, too—that somehow, this was a karmic punishment to be meted out for her past addiction to nicotine and her lack of willpower. This type of thinking is, simply, the anxious mind's attempt to "connect the dots" and to make sense of things. Human beings thrive on linear understanding, so Michelle's conclusion, while irrational, is not so difficult to understand when we consider the human discomfort with coincidence and randomness and the human tendency to make the coincidental causal. Being overly "scrupulous," or rigidly obsessed with issues of right and wrong or good and bad, is a subset of obsessive compulsive disorder (OCD),and a moralistic type of anxious thinking.

Media Exposure

The comedian Lewis Black quipped that once, while on a long flight, he read a 30-page magazine article about diabetes, and by the time the plan landed, he had diabetes. As often with humor, there is an element of truth in the joke: the more we are exposed to stimulus, the more susceptible we become to its influence. The news cycle is often fraught with frightening medical information. From recalls of everyday foods we purchase in supermarkets to novel strains of deadly diseases to household products that cause cancer, we are inundated with stories about how unsafe we are and how constantly threatened our physical health is. We are surrounded by warnings, cautionary tales, and stories of tragedy; it is part of the patchwork of our society. Overexposure to this type of information can cause us to become persistently worried, overly cautious, and avoidant and can grow into disordered thinking and disruption of our daily lives.

Vicarious Trauma

An underreported fact is that many medical professionals actually suffer with illness-related anxiety and worry. It stands to reason: the more a person is surrounded by illness, disease, and death, the more they may think about it and, perhaps, internalize it. According to a 2022 study by the Centers for Disease Control and Prevention (CDC), 22% of healthcare workers reported anxiety and post-traumatic stress as a result of their jobs.[10] This type of "vicarious trauma" imprints itself by turning what we witness inward, convincing us that it will befall us and that we are helpless to stop it. Jason, for example, was affected by the vicarious trauma of witnessing his coworker's heart attack.

Suppressed/Repressed Emotions

Suppressed or ignored feelings are similar to an overstuffed closet. Eventually, the door will no longer be able to close. Such is the case with the pent-up feelings that we push down or ignore; eventually, they will need a way to break free. Feelings like repressed anger and unprocessed grief can manifest physically in a variety of ways and in many of the same places where serious medical issues arise, leading us to believe that we are experiencing a more dire health problem. Centuries ago, philosopher René Descartes theorized that pain has a connection to the soul. This conclusion remains relevant today.

Extenuating Life Circumstances

Because illness anxiety can focus on and cause us to fixate on a single symptom, we often lose sight of the larger circumstances surrounding our lives. Countless life events and transitions can bring about feelings of uncertainty and anxiety from the joyful (getting married, having a child, etc.) to the somber (experiencing the death of a loved one, losing one's job, divorcing, etc.), and all bring with them complicated feelings and emotions. When we ignore the larger view of our lives, we often unduly and narrowly focus on one issue or symptom and become prone to unhealthy fixation. When we are anxious it is helpful to ask ourselves what else is happening in our lives that may be contributing to the body's physical response.

Geographic and Demographic Circumstances

Samantha grew up in a heavily industrialized area of her home state. When, in her 50s, she developed cancer, she was convinced that growing up around factories, refineries, and air and water pollution had played a role in her illness. History provides multiple examples of the environmental impact on illness, from Love Canal to Three Mile Island to other factory towns that have developed cancer clusters. Living in areas that are polluted, heavily industrialized, or otherwise environmentally compromised can increase not only real exposure to illness but also health-related anxiety and worry.

Samantha recalls living beneath high-voltage power lines and a block away from a large factory and its smokestacks. She recalls, too, feeling constantly worried about the environmental effects on her health and the health of her children. For those living in industrialized areas without access to nature, the inherent worry about their physical health and safety is difficult to escape. In social work, it is important to always consider the person-in-environment perspective when we look at problems such as anxiety and why it affects some individuals more strongly than others. We must also bear in mind that a disproportionate number of low-income and minority Americans live in these types of areas, which directly affects these populations' tendency to experience health-related anxiety.

Social/Biological Trends

In the early 1990s, after a story aired on the *Oprah Winfrey Show*, a widespread fear of Mad Cow Disease, which had claimed the lives of a number of children, swept across the United States. After highly publicized cases of *E. coli* infection, people also became paranoid about consuming contaminated meat and eating at fast food restaurants, particularly the West Coast chain Jack in the Box, where a number of the cases had occurred. "Societal anxiety," which can affect entire regions or countries—or, in the case of the COVID-19 pandemic, large parts of the world—can occur in the wake of outbreaks, epidemics, or pandemics.

Many individuals who did not previously experience health anxiety or "germaphobia" developed such fears in the wake of COVID-19. A flood of constantly changing, and sometimes contradictory, public health information resulted in heightened anxiety, uncertainty, and fear as the pandemic unfolded. While some of these fears were legitimate, it was not difficult to find oneself overwhelmed by crippling anxiety that illness and death were, in some ways, inescapable. This, naturally, led some people to engage in hypervigilant behaviors that negatively affected their daily functioning. If we view the pandemic as a worldwide trauma, then an escalation in health-related anxiety and hypervigilance is easily understood. The influence of social health cases and trends must be considered in the discussion of IAD, as widespread fear and irrational paranoia can result from the dramatic reporting of such incidents.

Natural Aging Processes

The older we get, the more our bodies become susceptible to discomfort and injury. The activities we used to do easily and without pain may, as we enter middle age, cause muscle strain, aches and pains, and other forms of physical discomfort. This increased vulnerability brings with it an increased sense of worry regarding our overall physical health. Common ailments related to aging such as muscle pulls or pinched nerves can be easily misinterpreted as more serious medical problems. It is important to understand the physical impact of the natural aging process, to adapt and adjust our level of physical activity as we age, and to understand that certain physical responses are purely the result of natural physiological processes and not indicators of a serious physical problem.

Existential Anxiety/Depression

According to data from the CDC, nine of the ten leading causes of death in the United States in 2021 were some form of illness or disease.[11] Deaths by natural causes are, overall, somewhat uncommon, so from a young age, we become accustomed to witnessing disease, failing health, prolonged illnesses, and complicated deaths. This embeds itself into our psyche, and, as is natural for humans, we cannot help but look inward and wonder and fret about our own mortality and physical longevity. While these thoughts are natural and common, too strong a fixation on our eventual atrophy and demise can lead to a heightened and constant sense of fear, anxiety, and existential dread.

Depression and anxiety are closely related; we might consider anxiety to be "hyperactive" (overactive), and depression to be hypoactive (underactive or lethargic). Interestingly, each can contribute to the other: enough hyperactivity can cause us to become tired, exhausted, and lethargic, whereas enough hypoactivity can leave us feeling uneasy, worried, and anxious. When we feel overwhelmed by thoughts about the purpose of life or depressed with feelings of hopelessness, we experience a vague yet overwhelming fear that can manifest through anxiety attached to different parts of our existence, commonly to our physical health or sense of personal safety (Figure 1.2).

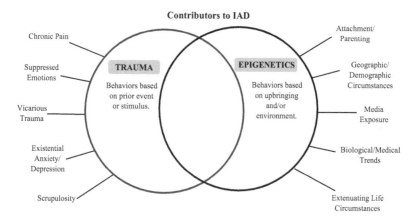

Figure 1.2 Venn diagram illustrating how trauma and epigenetics influence illness anxiety disorder.

IAD and Daily Functioning

One of the criteria that must be met for any psychological disorder is that it must negatively impact one's daily functioning. For some, the disruption in daily functioning is blatantly obvious (Colin left college as a result of his illness anxiety). For others, its manifestation is less visible. Jason would surreptitiously check his body for changes, keeping an oximeter in his pocket to allow him to check that he was getting enough oxygen. He would schedule medical appointments for before or after working hours without notifying his wife. Common to both patients was a decreased capacity to be "present" in their daily lives, with their attention often narrowly attuned to health-related concerns. This unhealthy fixation on possible medical problems can, in severe cases, border on obsession. Colin, even during early therapy sessions, would often run his fingers along his neck to feel for swelling or glandular changes that might signal a deeper medical problem.

Anxiety tends to narrow our view and, therefore, our world at large. The agoraphobic, for instance, narrows their existence to such an extent that they confine themselves to one house or even one room in an attempt to avoid possible disaster. Colin narrowed his life by leaving college; Justin, by filling space and time with booking and keeping medical appointments and traveling for tests, scans, and procedures. Healthy daily functioning allows us to care for ourselves (personal hygiene, exercise, hobbies, etc.), to honor our obligations (work, school, clubs, etc.), and to have space for our personal commitments (spouses, family, children, etc.). Anxiety robs us of one or more of these, leading to impaired daily functioning. Illness anxiety may cause a deeper loss; if a person is afraid of suffering a heart attack, for example, they may let go of healthy interests that they fear may exacerbate symptoms, such as exercise or cardio. Time spent researching symptoms or scheduling and attending medical appointments can cut into leisure time or time once reserved for pleasurable activities or social connection and engagement with others.

Many other areas of our lives that can be negatively affected by IAD. When we worry, we often experience disrupted sleep, difficulty with digestion, aches and pains, neglected diet, and impaired focus and attention. Any of these can contribute to a deficit in daily functioning and can have a marked impact on one's ability to be fully engaged in work, school, or family and social responsibilities. When daily functioning and ability to engage in required daily activities are affected, it is important that mental health treatment be sought.

Areas of Daily Functioning That Can Be Negatively Affected by IAD

- Personal hygiene (dental care, bathing/washing, shaving, etc.)
- Work duties (calling out sick, lack of focus on work-related tasks and obligations, leaving or missing work for anxiety-based medical appointments/visits to urgent care centers, etc.)

- Diet changes (overeating or undereating, restricting diet, poor dietary choices, etc.)
- Household obligations (care of pets, house cleaning, financial duties, etc.)
- Self-care (exercise, mental health activities, hobbies, etc.)
- Interpersonal relationships (alienation from and avoidance of social settings, isolation from others, fissures in marriages and relationships, difficulties with parenting, etc.)

Stress and the Body

Because they are responding to physical symptoms and discomfort, IAD patients often initially end up in medical settings rather than in mental health settings. Thus, there is typically first an investigation into the symptoms through exams, tests, and scans before the eventual conclusion that the symptoms may be due to stress or anxiety. This is often a difficult answer for the patient to accept, as it is somewhat vague and not easily translated to an immediately applicable treatment. Some patients will push against this conclusion, convinced that there must be an underlying physical problem. Again, this is not a manipulative response nor is it a patient "abusing" the healthcare system; rather, it is a fear-based response. What the patient wants more than anything is a clear answer that will allay their fears, and "stress" is not always received as a clear, concrete, or measurable explanation.

We have a deeper understanding of the body's responses to anxiety and stress than we once did. No longer do we see pain as simply a response to an injury or a purely physical phenomenon, separate from our emotions. Rather, we now understand that the physical and emotional systems work both with and, at times, against one another. We may view the body as a series of systems that work together to create an overall healthy organism. When one system falters, warning signs are disseminated throughout the larger system. The complication is that sometimes, these warning signs are tripped when there is no underlying emergency or problem—a reaction similar to a home alarm system being set off when there is no intruder. Often, when the emotional system and the physical system are misaligned, the signals that we feel in our bodies are difficult to understand and, therefore, easy to misinterpret.

We recognize now that overwhelm, stress, anxiety, and exhaustion can trigger our physical alarm systems as much as a physical injury can. Furthermore, the way they warn us is unique to the individual. Colin, for example, mainly experienced physical warnings in his neck, shoulders, and lumbar region, resulting in tightness and pain whereas Jason's warnings were mainly in his chest, resulting in heart palpitations and chest tightness. Other common areas of the body that carry these warnings include the gastrointestinal system, the cranial region, and the respiratory system. The problem for IAD patients is that these signals from these areas of the body can easily be misinterpreted. For example, a stress-induced headache may be misinterpreted by an anxious individual as a much more dire problem, such as a brain tumor or an aneurysm. Once this misinterpretation is arrived at, the anxious patient often tumbles headlong into worry and catastrophic thinking, resulting in the care-seeking and care-avoidant behaviors described earlier.

We understand now, too, that the body acts as something of a storage facility, remembering and housing past traumas. Our bodies can be hosts for disease and illness but also for frightening and traumatic memories. Michelle, who intimately experienced the slow and painful death of her mother from lung cancer, would report often experiencing shortness of breath and vague pain around her lungs. X-rays and CT scans would reveal that everything was normal, yet it was difficult for Michelle to accept. It was as though, through vicarious trauma, her body had learned to store her complicated feelings in the same physical region where her mother's body had housed cancer. As Michelle began therapy to process her complicated feelings about her mother's illness and death, and started a low dose of an antianxiety medication, her body slowly let go of its stored-up trauma. At some point, with enough processing and healing, the body forgets to remember (Figure 1.3).

STRESS IN THE BODY

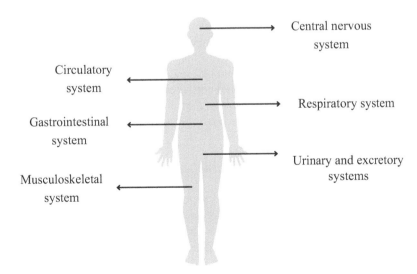

Figure 1.3 Image of the human body with arrows indicating different places in the body where people experience stress and anxiety.

Commonly Misinterpreted Physical Symptoms

The physical areas where anxiety manifests can be easily confused with serious medical emergencies and illnesses. If we felt anxiety in our toenails or hair follicles, we would most likely not draw catastrophic conclusions but when we feel it in our chest, our brain, and our stomach, it is more difficult not to think it may be something to worry about.

Muscle Contraction and Expansion

When we experience worry, stress, and anxiety, our muscles often tighten. When we consider how many of our anxiety centers are muscles, we gain a better understanding of why these areas respond so intensely when we are stressed. Understanding, for instance, that the bladder is a muscle may explain why many people report frequent urination when they are anxious. Similarly, some people may report diarrhea or lack of bowel control when they are nervous; recognizing that the rectum is a muscular tube explains this phenomenon. The heart, of course, is also a muscle, so it makes sense that it tightens and works harder when it experiences stress. The muscular systems' responses to anxiety, while frightening and intense, do not signal a larger medical emergency.

Organs and Cortisol

Cortisol is the body's naturally produced stress hormone. When it is triggered, it overproduces and focuses its distribution on the stressful feeling rather than on other necessary places, such as the immune system. During the stress response, cortisol is directed toward the organs, specifically the heart, resulting in escalated heart rate; the lungs, resulting in quickened breathing; and the brain, resulting in headaches, migraines, and brain fog. No wonder, then, that people experiencing anxiety often report a feeling that they cannot catch their breath, that their heart races, and that they are confused and unable to focus. These physical responses can be confused with serious issues such as heart attacks, aneurysms, or strokes.

Respiratory System

When we respond to fear, the body "battens down the hatches," preparing to preserve and protect itself. Rising blood pressure and increased respiration are the body's way of directing adrenaline toward its "fight" response. To the anxious person, this can cause feelings of lightheadedness, dizziness, and shallow breathing or shortness of breath as the respiratory system works harder and faster than it would in normal circumstances. These sensations can be easily misinterpreted as indicators of a medical emergency.

Central Nervous System

The central nervous system—in a sense, the switchboard of the body—works to receive and process sensory information and to disseminate signals to the body based on that information. When overwhelmed by sensory information, the signals that are sent out can negatively affect an individual's mood and emotions. For example, an overresponse to sensory information may cause the brain to flood the nervous system with hormones and cortisol, resulting in a physical response such as panic, and feelings of panic can easily mimic more serious physical problems.

When all of these systems (the various organ systems, the musculoskeletal system, the central nervous system, and the respiratory system) are overfunctioning at the same time, we often experience intense anxiety and panic as the body struggles to keep up with its system wide defensive fear response.

Symptom	Common Misinterpretation	Other Possibilities
Chest tightness/Heart palpitations	Heart attack/Cardiac emergency	Indigestion/Anxiety/ Depression
Headache/Migraine	Brain tumor/ Aneurysm	Eye strain/Tiredness/Dental or jaw problems
Frequent urination	Bladder disease	Nervousness/Anticipatory anxiety
Shortness of breath/ Lightheadedness	Seizure/Fainting spell	Panic attack/Asthma

Panic Attacks

One of the body's most intense responses to overwhelming emotion and stimulus is the panic attack. Ironically, in its attempt to alert us to danger, the body, by producing panic signals, frightens us more. Though different people experience panic in different ways, a general consensus regarding a panic attack is that it is scary and often feels as though one is losing control of oneself, "going crazy," or even dying. The connection to IAD is that panic attacks often mimic extremely serious medical conditions such as heart attacks, seizures, and strokes. Panic attacks cause many people to seek emergency medical care, only to feel OK by the time they are admitted to the hospital. They are later discharged with no answers and, often, a feeling of shame and confusion. One client reported being told by a doctor that he was "taking up a bed" by going to the emergency room for something that did not require immediate treatment. This type of clinical invalidation only worsens feelings of isolation and leads to further confusion as to how to cope and where to turn for answers.

Because the bodily responses during a panic attack are so heightened, the individual often has difficulty soothing or reassuring themselves. Rather, many people report being convinced that they are dying or experiencing a serious medical emergency. In the throes of a panic attack, it is nearly impossible to tell oneself that it is temporary or that it will last only a few minutes. Though it is true that physiologically, a panic attack will last approximately three to five minutes, its lingering effects are longer-lasting. In fact, many who have experienced a panic attack become anxious about the possibility of experiencing another one.

Panic attacks often leave individuals further confused and, therefore, more prone to seeking clinical answers. If, for instance, a person's panic attack manifested mainly in their chest and heart, they may seek out specialists such as cardiologists, take stress tests, wear heart monitors, and undergo numerous tests that ultimately reveal nothing amiss. Similarly, those who experience panic in the gastrointestinal tract may undergo tests of their stools and uncomfortable procedures such as colonoscopies and endoscopies. Of course, when appropriate, these tests can be helpful and necessary, but when fear-driven, they are often yet another layer of maladaptive care-seeking, that leaves patients answerless, frustrated, and more anxious.

Physical Symptoms of a Panic Attack

- Quickened heart rate/respiration
- Dizziness/lightheadedness
- Nausea/gastrointestinal discomfort
- Chest tightness/heart palpitations
- Feelings of confusion/disorientation
- Increased perspiration

Cognitive Distortions in IAD Patients

The IAD patient will exhibit a variety of cognitive responses to try to cope with their persistent fear and worry. Rather than simply viewing these cognitive patterns as "irrational," it is helpful to understand why they are used and what they intend to accomplish.

Catastrophizing/Awfulizing

The tendency of the anxious patient to "catastrophize" or to jump to the worst-case scenario is a way to protect themselves against a possible calamity. In the anxious mind, playing out the worst possible contingency is a cognitive attempt to cover all the bases in order to be prepared for any eventuality. The problem, however, is that this increases and escalates feelings of worry and impending doom and obscures the individual's ability to see the situation rationally.

Polarized Thinking

Also known as "all-or-nothing" thinking, this cognitive response sees things in an "only this" or "only that" form. For instance, an IAD patient may struggle to see any middle ground in a situation: a chest pain can *only* mean a heart attack, or a headache can *only* mean a brain tumor. This is a way for the individual to simplify the situation, but it complicates the reality by drawing an inflexible conclusion.

Overgeneralizing

When patients overgeneralize, they often make incorrect assumptions based upon a situation or stimulus. For instance, a patient who hears from a doctor that further tests are needed may overgeneralize this information and tell themself it means that something terrible will be found. This cognitive distortion takes specific information and turns it into general conclusions. Much like polarized thinking, this cognitive distortion is the individual's attempt to simplify a confusing situation. Ultimately, though, it is an incorrect oversimplification.

Emotional Reasoning

This is a form of thinking that downplays or ignores the rational side of things. When we base our conclusions purely on emotion, we are unable to view the more factual aspects of the situation. When feelings are interpreted as facts, we lose the ability to question conclusions driven by anxiety. When we are anxious, we often rely on and respond to our emotions, which prevents us from seeing situations rationally and logically.

Filtering

This is a type of thinking that focuses only on certain or filtered-out parts of a situation. A patient who receives a medical diagnosis, for instance, may fixate on the negative aspects of the diagnosis while ignoring the fact that their condition is treatable or manageable. Filtering is a selective, rather than a complete, attention to information. Filtering occurs because an anxious patient wants an answer above all else. But when they only process selective information, they ignore more reasonable or rational possibilities.

Accepting Anxiety as a Cause

When Corrine decided to adopt a gluten-free diet, she based her decision on her belief that she had irritable bowel syndrome (IBS). She would often experience gastrointestinal discomfort, diarrhea, and other stomach problems, particularly when she was stressed at her job. The feedback from multiple doctors had been that while they could not pinpoint anything in particular, IBS was a strong possibility. Accordingly, Corrine began to restrict her diet, removing any foods that could cause further gastrointestinal discomfort. In one instance, she was hospitalized for severe stomach pains. While nothing was found to be out of order, a hospital social worker visited her room and began asking questions about depression, anxiety, stress, and life circumstances. Corrine was confused as to why the focus had shifted from her physical symptoms to her personal life. Having never attended therapy, Corrine was unaware that there could be a correlation between her stress levels and her stomach issues.

Accepting anxiety, stress, and worry as causes of physical problems can be a challenge. Because our society is not necessarily skilled at psychoeducation, individuals often fail to make the connection between the emotional and the physical until all other medical investigatory options have been exhausted. When test after test comes back negative and visit after visit results in no concrete answers, the attention often shifts to the impact of stress and anxiety on the body. Once an individual accepts that the root of the problem lies in the emotions rather than in the body, they can seek appropriate mental health treatment and let go of overreliance on medical visits. But this acceptance does not come easily to all people: those who hold a stigmatized view of mental health services may be reluctant to begin psychotherapy or take antianxiety medications. The more we as a society work to normalize the physiological effects of stress and anxiety, the more we can prevent individuals from anxiously seeking unnecessary medical care.

The act of accepting is one of letting go of trying to figure it out. While understanding root causes is important, the real work in therapy is learning to navigate uncomfortable emotions and situations. Accepting that one has health-related anxiety and not a specific physical disease or illness can be freeing. It can allow a person to truly begin coping with and healing from their persistent, nagging feelings of worry and impending catastrophe. Anxiety and stress, while not observable through X-rays, scans, or blood tests, is often the reason behind more serious-seeming physical symptoms and, for the anxious patient, must be accepted as such so they can begin healing and moving forward with less worry.

The Medical Profession's Understanding of Illness Anxiety

We rely on doctors and medical professionals to keep us healthy. Often, we see them as supreme beings who hold all the answers to our physical concerns. But medicine, while obviously advanced, is not, and never will be, an exact science. Although there are general guidelines regarding health, each individual's personal health is unique and must be treated according to one's experience, genetics, life circumstances, and background. This is especially true for emotional health. Everyone's capacity to cope adaptively with life challenges is different and, unfortunately, the medical field does not always take this into consideration. Courtney, a healthy 30-year-old, saw a general practitioner for a routine checkup. While her vital signs were being taken, the nurse observed and mentioned that her blood pressure reading was high. Courtney had always felt nervous in doctor's offices—what some casually refer to as "whitecoat syndrome." While taking Courtney's vital signs, the nurse mentioned that her blood pressure reading was high, jotted down a note on her medical chart, and said nothing more. The nurse did not inquire if Courtney was anxious or provide any context or reassurance to her observation.

There are times, as in Courtney's case, when the medical profession can be so clinical that it can feel cold and detached and patients can be left feeling invalidated and shameful. Clinical empathy is as important as medical accuracy when it comes to a patient's overall sense of safety and well-being. Many doctors have excellent bedside manner and work to help their patients feel safe and understood; however, those who lack or underestimate this valuable trait risk contributing to their patients' anxiety and negatively affecting their overall health.

When Paul, a healthy 28-year-old, presented at the emergency department complaining of chest pains, the doctor on call commented, "What are you doing here? You're too young to be here." Paul felt immediately invalidated by this doctor's offhand remark. He felt, too, that he was not being taken seriously although his chest pains felt very real and caused him significant discomfort and worry. Despite his comment, the doctor did his due diligence and sent Paul for all the requisite tests, but Paul nonetheless suspected, that he was just being humored and he felt silly for having gone to the emergency department. Like so many other IAD patients, he was discharged from the hospital feeling not only answerless, but humiliated.

What can be done differently in the medical profession's approach to health-related anxiety? Foremost, an attempt to be both clinical *and* empathetic is paramount. An anxious person needs to feel safe, not ridiculed, minimized, or invalidated. Mental health screenings (performed through conversation with a provider rather than with a cursory self-reporting checklist) may also be helpful in addition to requests for information about a patient's emotional state. This will allow doctors to better understand a patient's emotions and to take them into consideration along with, rather than separate from, physical symptoms. Medical professionals can also offer education to their patients; for anxious people, understanding is an important part of coping. One client shared that after a cardiologist gently and patiently explained and demonstrated where different chest pains occur and what they mean, the client felt great relief and was more able to separate anxiety-based thoughts from more rational ones. Additionally, medical professionals should attempt to humanize and normalize feelings of health anxiety, as Chapter 2 will address.

Unhelpful Statements to Say to IAD Patients

- "It's all in your head."
- "Don't be a baby."/"Toughen up."/"Be strong."
- "You should google your symptoms."
- "You're fine."
- "You're too young for there to be anything wrong with you."
- "You're just being [ridiculous/irrational/dramatic/attention-seeking]."
- "Other people have real medical problems."

Sometimes, it is not the provider's approach that triggers a patient's anxiety but, rather, the larger medial system and how it functions. When Danielle, two months pregnant, noticed vaginal bleeding, she called her doctor and was instructed to get two rounds of blood work to be compared in order to determine if the pregnancy was viable or if she was likely to experience a miscarriage. Danielle's test results became available to her through her patient portal on a Saturday when her doctor's office was closed, meaning that she was able to view and interpret her results without guidance or information from her medical provider. Unbeknownst to Danielle, the lab had made an error; the information in the portal, which showed a significant drop in her hCG levels, suggesting a miscarriage, was incorrect. In response, Danielle did what most people in her situation would do as a response to what she saw: she went to the hospital. After waiting for five hours for a transvaginal ultrasound, she was assured that her results were incorrect and her pregnancy was healthy. Information is power, but information without proper guidance has the power to frighten us.

In the case of Danielle, we must resist the temptation to say, "All's well that ends well." Instead, we should pay attention to the emotional impact of medical misinformation; the system's failure to provide proper guidance; and its tendency to leave patients alone with test results and, therefore, with their own thoughts and interpretations of the information. The Hippocratic Oath, which instructs doctors to "first, do no harm," must also include the emotional and psychological harm that can be done by the medical system's tendency to leave patients on their own with test results and information. Danielle, pregnant for the first time at age 38, was already anxious about being pregnant at her age, and this experience, which easily could have been avoided, served only to increase her worry—not to mention, causing an unnecessary trip to the emergency room. A rethinking of the way certain aspects of the medical system function is pertinent to the discussion about illness anxiety and its preventable causes.

What the Medical Profession Can Do Differently

- Ensure that test and lab results are released with provider guidance.
- Provide accessibility to doctors outside of normal operating hours if lab results are made available to patients on nonworking days.
- Consider the emotional impact on a patient of releasing information without guidance.
- Work in tandem with labs to coordinate release of results and information.

Doctors, nurses, and other medical professionals save lives and keep us healthy. This is in no way meant to diminish their vital and invaluable work, only to point out that a combined understanding of physical and emotional health is important in ensuring proper patient care that truly "does no harm." There are many places within the profession and the larger system where this important confluence of the physical and emotional may be improved and strengthened.

Notes

1 American Psychiatric Association. (2022). *Diagnostic and statistical manual of mental disorders* (5th ed., text rev.). American Psychiatric Association.
2 Beck, A. T. (1991). *Cognitive therapy and the emotional disorders*. Penguin Books.
3 Freud, S. (1963). *General psychological theory*. Collier Books.
4 Almalki, M., Al-Tawayjri, I., Al-Anazi, A., Mahmoud, S., & Al-Mohrej, A. (2016). A recommendation for the management of illness anxiety disorder patients abusing the health care system. *Case Reports in Psychiatry, 2016*, 1–3. https://doi.org/10.1155/2016/6073598
5 Caron, C. (2022, October 29). Teens turn to TikTok in search of a mental health diagnosis. *New York Times*. www.nytimes.com/2022/10/29/well/mind/tiktok-mental-illness-diagnosis.html
6 Casanova-Perez, R., Apodaca, C., Bascom, E., Mohanraj, D., Lane, C., Vidyarthi, D., Beneteau, E., Sabin, J., Pratt, W., Weibel, N., & Hartzler, A. L. (2022, February 21). Broken down by bias: Healthcare biases experienced by BIPOC and LGBTQ+ patients. *AMIA Annual Symposium Proceedings, 2021*, 275–84.
7 From *Trauma and Recovery*. by Judith Herman, copyright © 1992. Reprinted by permission of Basic Books, an imprint of Hachette Book Group, Inc.

8 Wolynn, M. (2022). *It didn't start with you: How inherited family trauma shapes who we are and how to end the cycle.* Vermilion; Skinner, M. (2014). Environmental stress and epigenetic transgenerational inheritance. *BMC Medicine, 12*(153). https:// doi.org/10.1186/s12916-014-0153-y

9 Ravan, J. R., Chatterjee, S., Singh, P., Maikap, D., & Padhan, P. (2021, June 30). Autoimmune rheumatic diseases masquerading as psychiatric disorders: A case series. *Mediterranean Journal of Rheumatology, 32*(2), 164–67. https://doi.org/ 10.31138/mjr.32.2.164

10 National Institute for Occupational Safety and Health. (2022, May 11). *Health worker mental health.* Centers for Disease Control and Prevention. www.cdc.gov/ niosh/newsroom/feature/health-worker-mental-health.html

11 National Center for Health Statistics. (2022, December 8). *Mortality in the United States, 2021.* Centers for Disease Control and Prevention. www.cdc.gov/nchs/produ cts/databriefs/db456.htm#section_4

2 Coping with Illness Anxiety

Normalizing Health-Related Anxiety

Because our physical health and our possible acquisition of disease, illness, or injury are not wholly within our control, it is natural that we worry about them. Such is the case with anything out of our control; consider that more people fear flying (where someone else controls the vessel) than fear driving (where they control the vessel), though the statistics bear out that driving is significantly riskier. So, a sense of anxiety around our health and longevity is, to some extent, normal. Humanistic and existential psychology help us to understand that many of our "hang-ups" or "neuroses" are shared by a large part of the population. The maxim that there is "strength in numbers" holds some truth: the less we feel alien in our ways of thinking or our anxieties, the more we feel validated and allowing of our feelings, even those that are uncomfortable. Concepts like fear of death, uncertainty about the meaning of life, and the existence of God, for instance, are shared by many people across generations, geographical areas, and cultures. So, too, are worries about our health. There is healing and safety in commonality.

Often, though, we fail to see physical health through this humanistic lens, labeling those who worry about their health as "neurotic." Seeing with compassion and empathy, we understand that the prospect of becoming ill is, in actuality, quite scary. Furthermore, the realization that we will someday cease to exist is uncomfortable. There is a reason that Buddhist concepts such as "no death," which teaches us to accept death as merely a continuation of life, remain popular today; humans have wondered and ruminated about such mysteries for centuries. Many of our great works of literature and art are responses to these unanswerable questions. If we can begin to shift our rigid view of these topics as "bad," "taboo," "neurotic," or "verboten," we might see our feelings of discomfort as more normal and less something to feel shame or humiliation about.

DOI: 10.4324/9781032637921-2

Common Existential Fears

- Fear of abandonment
- Fear of loss of identity/purpose
- Fear of death/nonexistence
- Fear of becoming ill
- Fear of aging
- Fear of eternal punishment or damnation/not living up to moral standards

---

Internal and External Soothing

When we are little children and we have a scrape or a cut, our parents or guardians care for us; they know what to do and how to make us feel better. We trust them to help us heal. As adults, we are left to our own devices. But our need for external validation and soothing does not vanish simply because we grow into adulthood. Without an instruction manual on how to do it, we must learn to soothe ourselves when we are frightened or in pain. Societal messages, however, often impede our ability to do so. We are told to "toughen up," "keep it to ourselves," and "not complain." But asking ourselves what we need when we feel triggered and afraid is important to our ability to cope. It is no different than asking a parent to care for us when we are injured or sick. It is normal, not infantile or regressive, to feel that we need soothing. But the skill is to be able to provide it to ourselves as adults and to provide it in response to more vague "injuries" such as fear, worry, and stress.

External Soothing

We can receive external soothing and validation from multiple sources, including spouses and partners, family members, therapists, medical professionals, and others. What we must remember, however, is that we cannot *completely* rely on validation and soothing from eternal sources. As children, we had no choice but to depend on others to help us feel safe and secure; but as adults, this can comprise only a part of our overall sense of well-being. This highlights how care-seeking behaviors constitute an overreliance on safety and reassurance from external sources and an impaired ability to provide it to ourselves. When we over-rely on the "expertise" of others, we let go of our trust in ourselves and our own intuition. Those IAD patients who over-seek medical feedback are often simply looking for something to soothe their persistent sense of worry.

Internal Soothing

When we experience health-related anxiety, the message we often need to hear is that we are safe and healthy. This message does not necessarily need to be delivered by a doctor or medical professional. If we are not in an emergency situation, we can offer the message to ourselves. A simple and gentle mantra such as "I am OK" or "I am safe" can help us to self-soothe. Activities such as meditation, visualization, or deep breathing may help us slow down racing, anxious thoughts and, therefore, be less reactive or behaviorally responsive. When we feel soothed, we are more capable of viewing situations rationally rather than emotionally or impulsively. When we are soothed, we can healthily differentiate between emergencies and feelings of discomfort.

Way to Self-Soothe

- Employ mindfulness activities such as deep breathing.
- Engage in gentle, compassionate self-talk.
- Listen to calming music, peaceful sounds or white noise.
- Stretch, walk, or engage in light physical activity.

Self-Advocacy

Sometimes when we are at a doctor's office or hospital, we feel powerless and forget that in these circumstances, we still maintain some level of personal autonomy. After all, we know our bodies well; we've lived in them our entire lives. Our autonomy and power lie in our willingness to speak up and to advocate for ourselves. Releasing our feelings of shame around health anxiety can look like communicating to our healthcare provider that we feel nervous and asking questions or requesting that a provider give further information or more clearly explain complicated procedures, diagnoses, and examinations. Letting a nurse know, for instance, that often your blood pressure is higher when you are at a medical appointment may alleviate continued feelings of worry and reduce the emotional signal to the body to release more cortisol. It also "puts words around" feelings, which is often a way to feel relief from internal stress. Speaking our feelings is a form of self-advocacy that we always carry with us; the challenge, when we are anxious, is to remember to use it.

Another way we can advocate for ourselves is to be sure we understand the information and treatment we are being given. There are times when the sheer amount of information and the way it is presented can be overwhelming and confusing; we can feel lost in medical terminology and jargon. Asking questions if we feel unsure and not feeling embarrassed about requesting further information is vital in ensuring that we feel confident and comfortable about our treatment and in reducing anxiety.

Ways to Advocate for Yourself at Medical Appointments

Ask Questions

Confucius reminds us that "he who asks a question is a fool for a minute; he who does not ask is a fool for life." While asking for clarification might cause us to feel momentarily vulnerable or uncomfortable, it is, in the long run, helpful in attaining a complete understanding of our health status and treatment. When it comes to understanding your health, there are no silly questions.

Take Notes

Do not be hesitant to write down what your doctor is saying and to take notes. It is common to leave medical appointments feeling overwhelmed by the information and having difficulty remembering everything that was said or recommended. Whether you bring along a notepad or use a notetaking app on your cell phone, jotting down important information is a way to feel you have a clear understanding of your health.

Bring a Supportive Person

If you feel you might miss important information or forget to ask questions, it is acceptable to bring along a trusted person to support you and to ask additional questions or take notes for you. You may also elect to sign a consent form allowing your medical provider to share pertinent treatment information with another trusted party such as a spouse or family member. Further, bringing a person you trust can help you feel less anxious and more supported.

Request Clear Follow-Up Information

At the conclusion of your appointment, be sure you have a clear understanding of what you are expected to do next, whether that entails follow-up tests or future appointments. If the office does not provide one, you have the right to request a printout or follow-up email outlining information regarding next steps. This can help you feel you can stay cognizant of your health.

Understand Your Rights to Your Personal Medical Information

All patients are entitled to their personal health information (PHI). By definition, your PHI includes complete medical and clinical notes from your visits and all treatment and diagnostic information and documentation. Keep in mind that you are permitted to request any and all of your PHI from any of your medical or mental health providers and that your providers have an ethical and legal responsibility to provide it to you at your request. Under the Health Insurance Portability and Accountability Act (HIPAA) regulations, your PHI is considered protected information that only you and your provider have access to, unless you consent for it to be shared with another party.

Ensure That Your Provider Understands Your Mental Health

If you are anxious or struggle with depression or other mental health problems, make sure that your medical provider is aware of your concerns and of any other professionals you see or medications you take. A simple comment like "I wanted to let you know that I have been diagnosed with generalized anxiety disorder" or "I wanted to share with you that I sometimes experience anxiety at these types of appointments" can help your doctor in understanding the best way to treat you and to communicate medical information without causing you further anxiety.

Build a "Care Team"

Having a team of medical providers with your consent to communicate with one another can ensure that you feel supported and that all your concerns are being addressed by the appropriate professionals. This care team can include medical professionals, physical and occupational therapists, mental health professionals such as psychotherapists and psychiatrists, caseworkers, and others.

Triggers and IAD

Just like our brains, our bodies have memories. When traumatic or unpleasant memories are stored within us, they can be activated unexpectedly by unrelated stimulus. Consider the war veteran who is thrown into a panicked state when he hears loud fireworks because they sound similar to gunshots. Such is the case with stimulus that triggers our illness anxiety. When our bodies feel sensations similar to those that have caused us pain or fear in the past, our response is much like that of the war veteran. It is important to know our triggers; this knowledge helps us to prepare for them and to cope when they are activated. The veteran may know that, come July 4, he will likely experience discomfort. Therefore, he can prepare and care for himself when his triggers are activated. In the case of the IAD patient, this may mean an awareness of where in the body their triggers are felt. Different parts of the body hold different emotions for different people.

For Jason, the triggers were most often felt within his chest cavity. When he would be exposed to uncomfortable stimulus related to the heart or to a heart attack, he would immediately feel a tightening in the chest, heart palpitations, and an accelerated heart rate; everything would begin to feel like it was moving quickly. The trigger could be activated by a movie scene of a character suffering a heart attack or even by an overheard conversation about heart health. It was important for Jason to understand his triggers and, more importantly, to understand where they originated and why they were so intense. His up-close exposure to his colleague's fatal heart attack had embedded itself into his body's stress response, manifesting in the chest- and heart-related sensations that became active when he was triggered. Once the trigger activated Jason's physical response, panic would often follow and internalize, leading to a belief that Jason himself was experiencing a heart attack.

What did Jason need to reduce the intensity of his body's response? In therapy, Jason and his therapist worked on creating a "triggers action plan" to help him conceptualize ways to soothe himself when he was feeling triggered. Once Jason understood his triggers, their underlying cause, and the response within his body, he became able to prepare for them, recognize their appearance, and respond in a positive way without escalating to panic or an anxiety-based impulsive response.

Facts About Triggers

- Triggers are not predictors of future harm or risk.
- Triggers, while intense, cannot cause any actual physical harm.
- Triggers remind us of previous uncomfortable or frightening situations, and our bodies react as they did in the previous situation.
- Triggers can occur with or without warning.

Caregivers and IAD

Those who care for sick family members may be more prone to illness-related anxiety based upon the sheer proximity to illness and the personalized nature of caring for a closely related individual. This feeling is similar to being a first responder. Caregivers are often on the "frontlines" of helping their loved one manage their illness. Being a frontline worker comes with its own trauma: a constant exposure to disease and sickness, as well as a need to always be vigilant for health changes, emergencies, or urgent situations. The caregiver is not immune to feeling threatened themselves by illness. In the impressionable brain, uncomfortable or frightening images and situations implant themselves. A caregiver who has witnessed firsthand the toll of a terminal illness may begin to fear a similar personal outcome, even without rational evidence.

Burnout and exhaustion can exacerbate anxiety. A family member who is, while working and taking care of other daily responsibilities, also caring for a sick person is prone to burnout and may be unable to take adequate care of themself or find needed time to rest. This deprivation can bring about increased feelings of worry or fear. This is complicated by the fact that, having seen a parent, sibling, or close family member suffer and, perhaps, succumb to a disease, the caregiver may begin to believe they are genetically predisposed to acquiring a similar illness. This can translate into IAD behaviors such as compulsive symptom-checking, hypervigilance, and unnecessary medical visits and tests. The caregiver may also begin to ruminate and fixate on such concerns, resulting in a depressive or hopeless emotional state.

Caregivers require care themselves, but finding time for self-care becomes difficult when the majority of their time is spent caring for someone else. But self-care and separation from the illness are necessary for maintaining a healthy life balance. It is important for caregivers to recognize that intense and constant exposure to illness can prove traumatic and can trigger internalized and vicarious feelings of fear and dread.

How Caregivers Can Care for Themselves

- Attend psychotherapy and/or join a support group.
- Ask for help from other family members or members of the care team. Delegate responsibilities.
- Engage in self-care and pleasurable activities.
- Take time off from work if necessary (see if you may qualify for a paid leave of absence by contacting your company's human resources department). Be aware of allowances made to caregivers by the federal Family and Medical Leave Act.
- Surround yourself with supportive people.

Seeking Help

When we are overwhelmed by anxiety and our daily functioning is seriously affected, it is important to seek professional help. This is complicated, however, by negative social messages and stigmas that tell us asking for help is weak and that we must not be a burden to others. Further, we are led to believe that only "crazy" or "mentally ill" people go to therapy or take antianxiety medications. This type of messaging only keeps anxious people feeling alone, isolated, and helpless.

Psychotherapy/Counseling

Psychotherapy can help to "humanize" a client and "normalize" their problems. Often, a client begins therapy feeling that they are somehow alien or broken but, through the building of a therapeutic alliance, begins to feel their problems are somewhat common to the human experience. Such is the case with IAD. Many people feel anxiety around their health; it is, perhaps, more common than recognized. Therapy can also help patients learn and build skills for coping with and navigating anxiety and panic. Psychotherapists trained or well-versed in cognitive behavioral therapy and similar interventions possess the necessary clinical skills to help an IAD patient learn coping mechanisms for health-related anxiety. Often, an anxious person experiences a sense of relief once they have made the decision to begin therapy. As they build a therapeutic relationship with a caring therapist, they begin to feel supported and less isolated with their anxiety.

Medication

Psychiatric medications such as selective serotonin reuptake inhibitors, anxiolytics, and benzodiazepines have been proven effective in the treatment of anxiety and panic. In the case of intense IAD that affects daily functioning, medication is an option that should be considered. Although there is still some misplaced stigma attached to taking medication for anxiety, it is a safe and effective option that can help an individual experience less daily anxiety and disruption of normal activities. Medications that treat OCD may also be considered for IAD treatment, as many of the impulsive behaviors related to IAD are related to OCD as well. It is important to seek out a knowledgeable pre-scriber if you are considering beginning an antianxiety medication. Scheduling an appointment with a psychiatrist or psychiatric nurse practitioner is a good first step in understanding if medication is an appropriate treatment option for an IAD patient. How to approach and begin therapy and medication will be further explored in Chapter 3.

Support Groups

There is a saying within the psychology field: "Peer support is the best support." Indeed, feeling that you are not alone with your problems can promote healing and hope. With a little research a person can locate support groups, both in-person and online, where they can become a part of a circle of people who uniquely understand their circumstances. This commonality and community can help individuals to feel less isolated.

Group dynamics may be more casual or more clinical, depending on what a person is looking for. Many outpatient mental health clinics offer group therapy sessions that are facilitated by mental health professionals and are places where people can learn new and effective ways to cope with anxiety.

Treatment Approaches for IAD

After six months on leave, Colin returned to college with a renewed sense of safety in his physical health and a feeling that disaster no longer lurked around the corner. He had not forgotten what happened in the airport, but it no longer occupied such a large emotional and cognitive space. In therapy, a combination of theoretical approaches was helpful to Colin in recovering from his crippling anxiety. Often, a single intervention is too narrow to address all of the presenting and underlying issues related to IAD. Below are some therapeutic treatment approaches that may be helpful in treating patients with IAD.

Cognitive Behavioral Therapy

CBT is perhaps the first-line treatment of anxiety disorders, including IAD. Because it teaches clients to question and challenge their anxiety-driven conclusions, it allows for building evidence to discredit the anxious thought. In simple practice, it may look like this:

Event: Client experiences chest pain.
Automatic Thought: "I am having a heart attack and I need to call 9-1-1."
Challenge to Automatic Thought: "I am not experiencing any other phys-ical symptoms. I am also prone to heartburn, and I ate something spicy at lunch."
New, Adaptive Thought: "I am most likely not experiencing a heart attack and this physical discomfort I feel is likely unrelated to a heart attack and. It is more likely that I am experiencing indigestion. At this moment, I probably do not need emergency services."

This type of "thought-stopping" and challenging, the cornerstones of CBT, can help a client to slow down the rush and flood of thoughts that occur following an unexpected and uncomfortable physical symptom.

Rational Emotive Behavioral Therapy

An offshoot of CBT, REBT focuses on the "unconditional acceptance" of our-selves, our lives, and our situations through a rational, rather than an emotional, lens. REBT teaches clients to "dispute" irrational thoughts in the service of arriving at a more sensible, logical view of a situation. Because anxious cog-nitive patterns often lack logic, REBT is helpful in restoring and promoting a healthier, alternative way of looking at a situation.[1]

Dialectical Behavioral Therapy (DBT)

DBT helps patients find a cognitive "middle ground" between the emotion-driven mind and the logic-oriented mind. Because anxiety is most often emotion-based, it tends to ignore logic and rational thinking. This single-mindedness can result in unhealthy behavioral responses. Learning and implementing DBT skills can assist clients in tolerating feelings of discomfort rather than having to react emotionally to them. In the case of IAD, if a client learns to slow their cognition following an uncomfortable feeling, they have a greater opportunity to utilize logic to arrive at an appropriate behavioral response. For the IAD patient, this may mean the difference between seeking unnecessary emergency care and having a more reasonable response, such as scheduling a doctor's visit in the near future. DBT teaches clients to work and respond from their "Wise Mind," the healthy overlap of the emotional mind and the rational mind.[2]

Somatic Therapy

The word somatic, from the Latin for "of or pertaining to the body," refers to anything body-related. Somatic therapy is an umbrella concept that includes a number of body-based interventions such as meditation, yoga, physical exercise, dance or movement therapy, breathing exercises, and massage. Somatic therapy highlights the importance of the brain–body connection and should be considered as an option to help those struggling with IAD. Generally, somatic therapy skills can be taught to a client by a therapist or counselor.

Mindfulness-Based Cognitive Therapy (MBCT)

It is a Buddhist belief that anxiety "lives in the future," and the importance of mindfulness and presence in the moment cannot be overstated in the treatment of IAD. Mindfulness teaches clients to replace "what if" with "what is." In the case example given earlier, "what if" sounds like "My chest feels tight and that means I'm going to have a heart attack," whereas, "what is" sounds like "My chest feels tight right now in this moment." The "what is" thought is simply an acknowledgment of what is happening, without an attached assumption or conclusion. Through acknowledgment of our feeling in the moment, we are able to "be with" our feelings rather than respond emotionally or behaviorally to them.

Narrative Therapy (NT)

Narrative therapy teaches us to view our lives as a story but cautions us against focusing on only one part of the story. Often, we become singularly focused on the "problem story," the part of the larger narrative influenced by our challenges and problems. NT urges us to take a broader, more inclusive view of our life story, noticing and honoring both the problematic and challenging parts as well as the more comfortable and victorious sections. Through this approach, we begin to see our personal narratives as nuanced rather than one-dimensional. For an anxious person, anxiety loosens its grip and becomes only a portion of the story, not the entire story.[3]

Imaginal Exposure Therapy

Visualizing and imagining the situations that frighten us can be helpful in beginning to feel safe again and can promote a gradual return to activities and situations that have caused anxiety or avoidance. For example, a therapist may guide a care-avoidant client through an imagined scenario in which they have a medical visit at a doctor's office. Because the visualization is being done with the safe confines of the therapy office, the exercise may begin to rebuild safety and comfort within the anxious client's mind regarding the situation, promoting an eventual return to the actual situation. Once the client can visualize safely returning to a previously feared situation, they often can return to the situation in real life.

In Vivo Exposure Therapy

(Disclaimer: Exposure therapy should be used with caution and a mental health provider should ensure that this approach will not exacerbate a client's anxiety or fear.) "In vivo" is Latin for "in a living organism," and in vivo therapy is the act of a feared stimulus being reincorporated into an individual's life. For some clients, going directly toward rather than avoiding, the frightening stimulus can provide a renewed sense of safety and facilitate the recovery process. In the case of a person who has become hypervigilant about germs in the aftermath of the COVID-19 pandemic, for instance, a slow and safe return to everyday activities such as grocery shopping or eating in a restaurant may help rebuild sense of safety. As a person reexperiences some of the previously avoided activities, they may begin to feel safe and be able to reengage with a reduced level of anxiety and worry.

Psychodynamic Therapy

Psychodynamic therapy helps us to view a client's behavior through the lens of the person's past and the events they have experienced, particularly those from their childhoods. This way of looking at a client's behavior allows us to better understand root causes and reasons for particular behavioral responses. We see the situation through a broader lens that includes past events that may have an influence on current problems. If, for example, a client's parent was a germophobe, the client's psyche may have embedded this message, leading to an irrational fear of germs or illness. Understanding the origin point of the phobia or anxiety is helpful in beginning to unravel it and loosen its grip on the individual. This approach also helps us recognize that not all embedded trauma occurs through abuse or war; some traumas result from inconsistent parenting; adverse childhood experiences; and parents' own anxieties, phobias, and beliefs about the world.

Psychoeducation

Because anxious patients are often on a search for medical answers, providing them with education about anxiety, its causes, and its physical manifestation can be helpful in removing some of the uncertainty that comes with anxiety. When a patient understands why physical symptoms are occurring, they often report a reduction in the symptoms, or, at least, a reduction in cognitive fixation on the symptoms. When a patient understands how anxiety works, they often begin to feel that through this improved understanding, they can better manage and cope with these feelings.

Scarcity and Excess as Anxiety Responses

People who are frightened about their personal health status may become overly restrictive, carefully counting calories or sodium content or forcing themselves to exercise more than their body needs as preventative measures to guard against the possibility of illness. On the one hand, scarcity can be anxiety-based when it takes the form of deprivation. A person who severely limits their food intake due to an irrational fear of acquiring diabetes or becoming overweight may also undermine their body's ability to receive the proper amount of nutrients. On the other hand, excess can look like an overresponse to a perceived danger. A person who exercises multiple times a day every day of the week to ward off diseases caused by sedentary lifestyles may actually be taxing their body to an unhealthy degree, resulting in exhaustion or injury. Scarcity and excess, as anxiety responses, are two sides of the same coin: they are both overly vigilant responses to an imagined danger.

It is helpful to ask ourselves if our behavior is fear-based. When we respond behaviorally to anxiety, it often takes an all-or-nothing form. For example, a person who fears something bad happening decides they will *never* leave the house, while a person who fears something in the house will go wrong decides they need to be out of the house as *often as possible*. Both are hypervigilant overresponses to an anxious feeling. IAD can take a similar form: the patient goes all the way left or all the way right with little to no middle ground. The patient sees the doctor as often as possible or not at all. This style of thinking leaves no room for flexibility or mental agility, both of which are necessary to humans living complicated lives in a complicated world. Our ability to reassess, to pivot, and to change direction is essential for our health. When we speak of pain management, for instance, a willingness to "figure it out as we go" is vital, noting what works and what doesn't, what reduces the pain and what increases the pain, all in the name of feeling as comfortable as possible.

There can be, too, a movement toward excess in the name of resignation. Jerry, after suffering a brain tumor that left him paralyzed from the waist down, began smoking cigarettes again though he'd quit the habit decades earlier. In his mind, it didn't matter; he had lost a large part of his health so smoking was not going to do much more damage. This type of behavior can be another side of care-avoidance. Not only is care avoided in the name of resignation, sometimes, additional self-inflicted pain and risk are layered on top of the illness in the form of maladaptive coping.

Cyberchondria and Self-Diagnosis

Our search for answers has never before been so easily and instantly gratified. The Internet affords us the ability to research practically anything at any time—for better or worse. If you search "left arm pain" on Google, for example, three immediate results will follow, one of which is that it is a sign of a heart attack, following "bone or joint injury" and "pinched nerve." The anxious mind will naturally gravitate toward the most catastrophic option, fixating on heart attack rather than pinched nerve or joint injury. This example helps us understand how the Internet can contribute to health anxiety. In addition to the accessibility of information is the tendency to self-diagnose, with our diagnoses often based on not necessarily reliable information found online. Though not recognized by the DSM-5, "cyberchondria" (a play on words combining "cyber" and "hypo-chondria"), or phobias developed and worsened through repeated, maladaptive Internet searching of medical information, is certainly on the rise. This type of "armchair diagnosis" only serves to escalate anxiety. When we research phys-ical symptoms online, we are not receiving a personalized response; rather, we are seeing overly generalized information that may or may not apply to our unique physicality and makeup.

With the increased accessibility has come increased confusion, as we can find ourselves overwhelmed by the sheer amount of information available to us. How, when our search results may yield everything from "normal pain" to "seek immediate medical attention," could we not find ourselves overwhelmed and confused? Any medical information found online should be vetted and the source considered with great scrutiny. As reputable as a website or informational source may be, it is not a replacement for personalized medical care. We need to be mindful not to confuse the *accessibility* of information with its *applicability*.

Self-diagnosis is a growing concern among the medical profession. Just a few clicks on a website can result in a full-blown diagnosis of ourselves, both physical and psychological. The danger with self-diagnosis is that often, we are broadly applying criteria that, to be truly accurate, should be applied more specifically. For instance, a person who sometimes gets distracted is not necessarily a candidate for a diagnosis of ADHD. Similarly, a person who experiences persistent headaches is not necessarily a candidate for a diagnosis of a brain tumor. But the Internet often creates the appearance and illusion of these diagnoses being not only accurate but also immediately applicable and conclusive. Viewed rationally, self-diagnosis or personal medical conclusion is nothing more than a guess. As with any other hypothesis, a self-drawn medical conclusion requires further evidence before it can be accepted as true. The appeal of self-diagnosis, however, is its immediacy in providing an "answer," even though the fact that the answer may be inaccurate. As humans, we are uncomfortable waiting to find out. When we are in pain or discomfort, we want to know what is happening, what it is called, and how to treat it. And this human desire can lead us down a slippery slope of Internet sleuthing, resulting in incorrect medical diagnosis and undue fear and anxiety.

Common Pitfalls of Online Medical Information

- Unreliable sources
- Overly simplified diagnostic information
- Generalized conclusions of complicated symptoms
- Anecdotal rather than clinical information
- Information not vetted by medical professionals
- Information shared by "influencers" rather than by medical professionals

---

Boundaries with online information are important—in a simple sense, knowing when to say "when." For instance, seeking peer support in online forums or groups can be helpful but, too deep a dive can lead to further anxiety and overwhelm. One IAD patient reported that at first, partaking in a Reddit group about illness anxiety was helpful, but after a while, it became overwhelming and triggering, making her anxiety even worse and creating more opportunities for drawing catastrophic, unlikely conclusions about her health.

Questions to Ask Yourself

- Is this information helpful to me, or is it causing me more worry and confusion?
- Are other people's stories triggering me or influencing my thoughts?
- Is everything I am hearing or reading applicable to my unique situation?
- Am I relying too much on online advice and information?
- Am I replacing verified information with anecdotal information?

- Am I spending an unhealthy amount of time researching and reading online information?
- Is my time spent researching detracting from other important life activities?

Coping with a Medical Diagnosis

What if, after all the anxiety, a person's illness-related fears come true? This happened to Richard, a 55-year-old schoolteacher who had spent the better part of a decade worrying that he would acquire a serious and possibly terminal illness. The day he was diagnosed with cancer, Richard felt somehow redeemed—while also terrified. His biggest fear had come true. He had finally gotten what he'd sought for such a long time: an answer to his vague worries about his health. But the answer came with its own worries regarding his prognosis, his recovery, his future, and his mortality. In this first therapy session following the diagnosis, Richard's therapist reminded him, "The goal of therapy was not that nothing would ever happen regarding your health, but, rather, that if it did, you would be able to navigate through it." Such is the case with anxiety: as much as we wish to never experience anything negative, it is only that—a wish. When we accept, no matter how long it takes us, that we are not immune to unexpected or frightening scenarios, we actually become free to view ourselves as relatively safe and capable of handling difficult circumstances if they should arise.

Richard, now three years in remission from cancer, no longer seeks constant reassurance through scheduling medical appointments, tests, and scans. Rather, he tries (with varying success) to look at his emotions rationally and to hesitate before responding behaviorally. While his brain and body remember the fear and anxiety of finding out his diagnosis, Richard is able to recognize that triggers that call back those uncomfortable feelings are neither predictions of future outcomes nor a return to the previous situation. Richard obviously never wanted to receive a cancer diagnosis, but when he did, he was well equipped with the skills to manage and navigate it. He follows up as instructed with his doctors and oncologist; he takes care of himself and his body, and he works to manage, through therapy and the coping skills he has mastered, feelings that veer back toward illness anxiety.

Notes

1 Ellis, A., & Ellis, D. (2019). *Rational emotive behavioral therapy.* American Psychological Association.
2 Linehan, M. M., & Linehan, M. (2015). *DBT skills training manual.* The Guilford Press.
3 White, M., & Epston, D. (1990). *Narrative means to therapeutic ends.* W.W. Norton & Company.

3 Recovering from Illness Anxiety Disorder

Trusting Our Bodies Again

In recovering from IAD, we must work toward trusting and paying attention to our bodies. We understand what happens when the signals are crossed, when the emotions and the physical body are at odds. We know how anxiety, panic, stress, and worry can blur reality and obscure what is really happening. Anxiety can tell us (believable) lies and convince us that we are in constant, serious danger. When we learn to trust our physicality, we let go of constant, anxiety-based surveillance of ourselves. We check less obsessively but still remain cognizant and aware of our condition and our health. We find middle ground, wherein we care adequately for ourselves but don't overdo it with constant hypervigilance or fear of worst-case scenarios. Further, we begin to listen to our bodies and trust that they will alert us of problems or concerns. If we listen without paying anxious attention, these signals cease to be alarm bells and hair-trigger smoke detectors and become more gentle reminders and indicators.

When, for instance, we experience a headache, we are able to consider slowly and rationally what is happening and what to do, if anything. Our anxious mind does not tightly grasp on to the first worrisome thought: "I have a brain tumor." Rather, it explores "what is" and not "what if." We are able to slow our automatic thoughts and be in touch with what is occurring in the moment. We are able to come to rational conclusions such as "I've been starting at a computer screen all day" or "I've had more caffeine than I typically do." We are, then, able to arrive at rational behavioral responses such as "I will take ibuprofen" or "I will step away from my laptop and reassess how I'm feeling in a little while." We are able, too, to recognize that there is no need for emergent, fear-based solutions such as rushing toward emergency care or hospitalization. We recognize that there are other actions that we can take first. A headache, or any other physical pain or discomfort is our body trying to tell us something. The skill is being able to listen without an anxious rush to judgment, conclusion, or impulsive action.

DOI: 10.4324/9781032637921-3

When we learn to trust our bodies, we once again feel safe. From that sense of safety grows self-trust and a belief that we will, most of the time, be OK—but also, that if something frightening or unexpected arises, we will be equipped and competent to handle it. In his book *Man's Search for Himself,* psychologist Rollo May writes of "a little girl coming home from school after a lecture on how to defend oneself against the atom bomb" and asking "her parent, 'Mother, can't we move someplace where there isn't any sky?'"[1] When we return ourselves to a sense of safety, we realize that anxious thoughts are merely part of the sky, like clouds; they are not the sky itself.

Restoration of Daily Functioning

When we heal from IAD, we also heal from anxiety-induced behaviors of hypervigilance, constriction, and numbing. We regain our ability to focus and be present; we are less fixated on physical symptoms, their meanings, or on trying to analyze them. We broaden our worlds and lives once again, letting go of avoidant behaviors and isolation. We rediscover healthy ways to cope when we are feeling uncomfortable or triggered. These rediscoveries culminate in a return to our previous level of daily functioning. Without hypervigilant fixation, we once again have room and capacity for our work, families, and social lives. When we no longer constrict ourselves, we open ourselves up to previously avoided opportunities and positive experiences. When we replace unhealthy numbing with healthy coping, we develop adaptive means of managing when things get overwhelming.

When we have the capacity for all the aspects and compartments of our lives, we are functioning at our optimal level. Areas that had been negatively affected fall back into place: personal hygiene and self-care, fulfillment of duties and obligations, appropriate time for leisure activities, and presence and participation in our daily lives. In healing from IAD, we regain a sense of safety, which allows us to live full and complete lives.

Signs of Restored Daily Functioning

- Fulfillment of work/school duties and obligations
- Ability to create a healthy work/life balance
- Positive social and personal relationships
- Restored interest in leisure activities and hobbies
- Proper attention to personal hygiene and self-care
- Appropriate seeking of medical care that is not anxiety-driven or impulsive

Colin

When Colin returned to college, he was able to resume the life he had temporarily left behind in the name of anxiety and care-seeking. He eventually finished his studies, graduated and is now living a "normal" young adult life. Colin's ability to bounce back is indicative of one of the unique traits of human beings: resiliency.

Jason

Jason, much like Colin, was able to heal from his illness anxiety. Over time, he let go of anxiety-based seeking of medical answers and reassurance. Therapy helped him process the trauma of witnessing his colleague's heart attack and develop new, healthier coping skills for anxiety.

Michelle

Michelle's recovery consisted of two intertwined parts: healing from the illness and death of her mother and learning new ways of coping with her fixation on herself acquiring a serious, life-threatening illness. As she accomplished this, her life returned to a more "normal" focus, with Michelle's attention placed back on her family, her work, and her life rather than on what-ifs or anxiety-driven possibilities.

When to Seek Medical Care

When patients are uncomfortable enough to seek out medical care, there is a fine line between doing so in a healthy (adaptive) manner and in an unhealthy (maladaptive) one. Repeated requests for care, making appointments, scheduling medical tests, and doctor shopping are forms of maladaptive care-seeking. All these actions are taken due to a patient's anxiety. For a person who feels frightened of a medical outcome, one professional's opinion may not set their mind at ease; they may seek a second or even a third or fourth opinion. This can involve going out of their insurance network and paying high out-of-pocket premiums or traveling inconvenient distances to find other providers. This may also result in duplication of services; multiple rounds of the same test or scan; and an overreliance on a doctor, their staff, or their office, not to mention significant financial strain.

If You Have Incurred a Large Medical or Hospital Bill

- Contact the medical office, facility, or hospital to inquire about payment plans.
- Contact your insurance provider to see if any of your out-of-pocket expenses may be submitted for possible reimbursement.

- Do not make any immediate payments if you have questions or confusion regarding what you are being billed for. Contact the medical office or hospital's billing department with your questions you may have.
- Research whether there are any state or federal aid programs that can assist you with making payment. You might start with your state's department of health.

Appropriate Care-Seeking

There are occasions when it is not only appropriate but also necessary to seek treatment or medical intervention. The IAD patient often has difficulty identifying these occasions. Physical symptoms are often difficult to pinpoint, so it can be challenging to tell the difference between something that requires immediate attention and something that can wait. Appropriate care-seeking is understanding when to seek medical advice in an urgent fashion and when to wait. One patient, who feared that he had undiagnosed heart problems, recounted a visit to a cardiologist in which the frustrated doctor commented, "I can't tell you what every physical sensation you have means." While the doctor's delivery and bedside manner leave something to be desired, the message is pertinent: it is not helpful or healthy to have an emotional or a behavioral response to every physical sensation we experience. If we do, we run the risk of overreacting to situations that, rationally, do not require a behavioral reaction. Often, this leads to unnecessary doctor's visits or unneeded medical tests.

Knowing when to seek care in an appropriate fashion is achieved only through an ability to respond to situations rationally rather than emotionally. While immediate feelings may arise when we experience physical pain, these feelings should not dictate what we decide to do next. For instance, an intense back pain may produce immediate fear. If we respond based on this feeling, we may seek emergency care. If we respond based on the symptom rather than the feeling, we may put a heating pad on our back, take a pain reliever, rest, and/or leave the option open to schedule a medical appointment if the pain persists for the next few days.

Tips for Appropriate Care-Seeking

- Try to differentiate between emergency and non-emergency situations.
- Follow recommended guidelines such as yearly medical checkups and physicals.
- Don't overschedule or overutilize medical testing or doctor visits.
- Don't avoid medical treatment or necessary preventative care measures.

Considerations for When to Seek Care

- The symptom or problem has been present for a significant length of time.
- The symptom has worsened or intensified significantly since onset.
- The symptom is causing daily disruptions to your quality of life.
- The symptom is the result of a known injury.
- The symptom has not responded to over-the-counter medications or at-home treatments.
- The symptoms are relevant to an illness to which you are genetically predisposed (e.g., a person with a family history of melanoma who notices a significant change in a mole on his body).

Differentiating Between Disease and "Dis-Ease"

Another way we might view how to arrive at appropriate care-seeking is to differentiate between "disease" (diagnosable symptoms) and "dis-ease" (feelings of uneasiness). In Buddhist philosophy, "dis-ease" is anything that causes us pain or suffering. While physical ailments can cause significant pain and suffering, so, too, do emotions such as anxiety, fear, and panic. When we are ill at ease, it can be difficult to distinguish between physical and emotional pain. Buddhist teachings go on to explain three types of dis-ease: "the suffering of suffering," "the suffering of change," and the "suffering of existence." All three are related to our emotions and circumstances, rather than to our physical health. In our effort to separate the uneasiness of being human from the uneasiness of a specific physical ailment, we can learn to pay close attention to our circumstances. If, for instance, we are stressed at work, overwhelmed, tired, and run-down, we may experience dis-ease that is not related to any physical problem. The key is to notice what else is occurring around us. When we ignore the circumstances, we can easily fixate on a single, misplaced anxious belief about our physical state.

Life Situations That Cause "Dis-Ease"

- Overwhelm at work/failure to create a healthy work–life balance
- Strained or difficult personal relationships
- Lack of sleep or inability to rest
- Overscheduling or stretching yourself too thin
- Taking on others' problems/people-pleasing
- Dehydration/poor diet/lack of attention to basic physical and nutritional needs

- Common life stressors (finances, work projects, childcare, etc.)
- Life transitions (changing jobs, buying a home, marriage/divorce, childbirth, etc.)

In the classic text *Zen Mind, Beginner's Mind,* Shunryu Suzuki extolls the virtues of "believing in nothing," explaining, "In our everyday life our thinking is ninety-nine percent self-centered. 'Why do I have suffering? Why do I have trouble?'"[2] Letting go of the need to attach a belief or a conclusion to every sensation we experience can allow us to let go of anxious thinking. We will never be fully without dis-ease, but we can live contentedly with the knowledge that not all uneasiness signals a larger, catastrophic problem and that in fact, much of our dis-ease is common to the human condition.

Grieving the Anxious Self

When we recover from anxiety, we are saying goodbye to a part of ourselves that has been in place for a long time. Although it is a loss that will ultimately help us, it can initially feel strange or uncomfortable. Any time we let go of something that we have held on to for a long time, we feel at first that we are losing part of our identity. Anxiety, however, was never truly a part of us; rather, it was a response to stimulus. What we are really saying when we let go of anxiety is "I am ready to respond to uncomfortable stimulus in a different, healthier way." Our initial emotional response to this letting go may be to feel incomplete. Ultimately, though, we may experience a feeling of great relief, freedom, and wholeness; a newfound meaning behind our experience; and a readiness to move forward.

The process of grieving does not follow a linear progression. Through more of a zigzag path, we may feel angry, sad, ambivalent, accepting, or in denial. When we grieve the loss of our anxious self, we may feel angry at it at times, sad to lose it at other times, and at still other times, happy and accepting. Allowing ourselves to experience these complicated, nonlinear emotions is important. This letting go or loss of something we have grown accustomed to ("everyday loss") is a radical change, much like adjusting to a physical death. It is accompanied by a mix of fluctuating feelings, all of which must be accepted and experienced in the service of healing and moving forward.

Mourning "Everyday Losses"

- Becoming accustomed to something no longer being there
- Accepting and embracing the "new" situation
- Deriving meaning from what you have lost or let go of

- Allowing yourself to feel mixed and complicated emotions related to the loss
- Reminding yourself that you are better off without what you have let go of

Self-Efficacy and Self-Trust

When we no longer rely solely on the feedback and reassurance of others, we build our own sense of self-trust. IAD can cause us to lose trust in our intuition and thus require constant reassurance from medical professionals. This can create a larger loss of personal autonomy, causing us to feel unsafe and constantly threatened. Regaining our sense of trust in ourselves allows us to think rationally and calmly about situations and to make proper decisions regarding how to proceed following intense or upsetting stimuli. A response to an uncomfortable physical symptom based in self-trust might sound like:

> I am experiencing chest tightness but I know that I have no underlying symptoms or preexisting conditions. I know, too, that I have had my yearly check-up and all was well. This is an uncomfortable feeling but there is nothing I need to do about it right this minute. I can monitor this in a calm way and reassess how I feel in a little while.

In this example, the individual relies on their ability to be cognizant and mindful of their health, without jumping to anxious or fear-based conclusions.

Distinct from self-esteem (how we feel about ourselves), self-efficacy relates to how we feel about our competency, our ability to handle situations, and our trust in ourselves. Self-efficacy means that we can be mentally agile, able to rationally assess and reassess situations as they occur and evolve. Anxiety keeps us mentally rigid, with little ability to see the nuance in a situation—hence the IAD-driven tendency to arrive at fixed, inflexible conclusions and behavioral responses related to physical symptoms. A mentally agile approach allows us to (1) notice what is happening, (2) decide if any immediate action is required, and (3) reassess the situation in a healthy, non-impulsive manner. Mental agility allows us to slow down and think rationally before going to the emergency department or jumping to an irrational conclusion.

Skills of Self-Efficacy

- Self-awareness: paying attention to thoughts, emotions, behaviors, and physiological reactions and observing them rather than judging them.
- Self-regulation: the ability to adjust our thoughts and behaviors according to a particular situation.
- Mental agility: the ability to view situations from different perspectives and to think flexibly.[3]

Self-Care and IAD

"Self-care" is one of those mental health buzzwords that we hear so often it almost becomes background noise. Even so, the importance of caring for ourselves as a way to reduce stress and anxiety cannot be understated. What many get wrong about self-care, however, is the idea that it is a radical act for which we must clear our schedules and spend loads of money. Self-care is not necessarily a day at an expensive spa or a luxurious vacation.

Daily Self-Care

- Adequate hydration and healthy diet
- Time spent moving the body/engaging in physical activity
- Firm and appropriate boundaries with work/work–life balance
- Time devoted to rest/leisure activities
- Space and time for social connections and relationships

The way that self-care affects anxiety can be viewed through the lens of childhood: think about what you needed when you were little and you experienced difficult emotions or a physical injury. Above all, you needed care. That care may have included nutrition, time for play, human connection, and rest, as well as comfort and safety. Seen this way, our needs haven't changed much since we were little, but the way it is provided to us has changed. It's on us now to know how to care for ourselves when we are injured, either physically or emotionally.

Self-Care Inventory

Rate each on a scale of 1 (lowest) to 5 (highest) to learn where you can devote more attention to your own care.

I drink enough water during the course of the day. 1 2 3 4 5

I make a consistent effort to make healthy food and diet choices. 1 2 3 4 5

I have a healthy relationship with my job/school, and I am able to create boundaries to maintain a healthy work/life balance. 1 2 3 4 5

I have outside-of-work hobbies and interests that bring me joy and that I do just for me. 1 2 3 4 5

I am able to engage in these hobbies and interests when I am stressed or overwhelmed. 1 2 3 4 5

I make a consistent effort to maintain strong and positive personal and social relationships. 1 2 3 4 5

It does not bother me to sometimes say "no," decline invitations, or let others know that I am not available. 1 2 3 4 5

When I feel tired or burned out, I allow myself to rest without feeling guilty. 1 2 3 4 5

I can be comfortable with being "unproductive" or engaging in an activity that does not have a direct outcome. 1 2 3 4 5

Healing Anxious Attachment and Inconsistent Parenting

In her book *Toxic Parents,* Susan Forward writes that "an unpredictable parent is a fearsome god in the eyes of a child."[4] Parental inconsistency can result in later feelings of anxiety and fear, generalized to one stimulus or more ambiguous and free-floating. Healing from this type of inconsistent parenting is important in once again feeling secure in our own lives. Being unsure whether or not we will receive soothing when we are afraid can generalize into our adult lives. When wounds, physical or emotional, are not tended to consistently by parents, we become conditioned to feel alone, isolated, and frightened when we are injured. This persistent fear can be a recipe for care-seeking illness anxiety.

"Inner child" and "reparenting" work are currently popular in psychotherapy for the very reasons described earlier. Learning, even as adults far removed from childhood, how to comfort our wounded selves is an important step in reducing persistent feelings of anxiety, isolation, and worry. When we learn how to soothe ourselves, we work to reverse longstanding emotional patterns of feeling unprotected and unsafe. As we do this work, physical symptoms that had been overwhelmingly frightening begin to feel less dire and threatening. Headaches no longer signal tumors; vague aches and pains no longer indicate some unseen physical malady. Knowing that we can care for and soothe ourselves works toward rebuilding a sense of safety in our lives and can help reduce anxiety related to becoming ill.

Ways to "Reparent" Ourselves

- Know what makes you feel happy and relaxed, and engage in those activities when it is helpful to you.
- Reengage in simple, joyful, even childlike activities that you may have gotten away from (reading, listening to music, playing games, doing puzzles, enjoying outside activities, etc.).
- Work to process through anger you may be holding on to from your childhood or related to the way you were parented.

- Form and maintain healthy relationships with others.
- Recognize that you are competent and capable of knowing how you feel, what you need, and how to provide yourself with caring and soothing.

Sitting with Uncertainty and Discomfort

Anxiety is unable to accept the fact that there will always be some level of uncertainty in our lives, no matter how planful or cautious we are. We simply cannot prepare for every eventuality. Anxiety bristles at this notion, arming itself against the unknown with heightened physical and emotional responses, confusing uncertainty with danger and conflating possibility with probability. When anxious people begin to accept that uncertainty does not necessarily equate to danger, they begin to feel more at ease. It is human nature to feel uncomfortable when we are unsure. But that does not mean we need to react to the feeling.

When we learn to differentiate between unpleasantness and unbearableness, we begin to recognize that we possess the ability to "sit with" our uncomfortable feelings. Anxiety is always uncomfortable, but it is rarely intolerable. Physical sensations such as muscle and joint pain, headaches, and gastrointestinal discomfort are unpleasant. When we experience these, we often want nothing more than to be rid of them. This can lead to a narrow fixation and focus on the symptoms themselves, which, in turn, heightens our feelings of anxiety and worry about them. Dialectical behavioral therapy teaches us to "ride" the discomfort, much like surfing a wave. If we can do this, we reduce fixation, which reduces our anxiety about the symptom.

In learning to tolerate discomfort, we neither react immediately or impulsively to an uncomfortable feeling, nor do we completely ignore it. Rather, we acknowledge and accept that it is there. Often, within this acceptance, we reach a peaceful and still point where we are not overwhelmed or driven by anxious or catastrophic thoughts. An IAD patient can learn to accept their feelings without needing to analyze them or draw anxious conclusions from them.

Starting Therapy or Medication

Beginning therapy can be daunting and make you feel vulnerable. But building a therapeutic rapport with a trusted and skilled therapist or counselor can help you feel supported. These professionals can also help you learn coping skills for uncomfortable feelings like anxiety and panic.

Differentiating Between Providers

Psychotherapists

These are mental health professionals who are credentialed and licensed to provide talk therapy. They may be licensed clinical social workers (LCSW, LMFT), licensed counselors (LPC, LAC, LMHC), or psychologists (PsyD). These professionals studied psychology/human behavior and completed graduate and/or doctoral programs.

Psychiatrists

These are medical professionals who specialize in psychiatric medicine and who can prescribe medications to treat psychological disorders, such as those related to anxiety. These individuals studied at medical schools and may be board-certified psychiatrists (MD/DO) or psychiatric-mental health nurse practitioners (PMHNP).

Tips for Finding the Right Therapist

- Research available providers in your area using your insurance provider's website and provider database or an online database such as *Psychology Today*.
- Schedule a consultation or a phone call/meeting before scheduling sessions. This can give you the opportunity to ensure that the provider is a good choice for you. Ask any questions you have about treatment, the provider's credentials and specialties, and their treatment approach. For IAD, therapists who are experienced in treating anxiety and panic, and skilled in offering behavioral therapy are typically a good fit.
- Determine if you have any preferences about your clinician such as their gender, age, ethnicity, sexual identity, or lived experience. Many clinicians will have this information listed on their online profiles, but if not, it is acceptable to ask.
- Decide if you plan to see a provider through your insurance carrier or if you will be paying for services out of pocket. If you are paying out of pocket, inquire about sliding scale agreements, where your therapist may be willing to negotiate a rate that is reasonable and fair to both parties. Also, be aware that you may be able to receive reimbursement for out-of-pocket payments by submitting paid invoices if allowed by your insurance carrier. You should contact your insurance carrier to determine if this is an option.

If you decide to explore a medication option, you will need to connect with a prescriber such as a psychiatrist or a psychiatric nurse practitioner. This type of professional can assist you in navigating a medication intervention that will be helpful in treating your presenting problem. Often, a combination of talk therapy and medication is effective in treating anxiety disorders.

Tips for Beginning Medication

- Be sure that you feel your prescriber has adequately described what to expect from the medication, including possible side effects and expectations about the timeline for noticeable positive change. You should understand and be comfortable with your provider's plan for your treatment.

- Try not to view taking medication as a "failure" or "weakness." Rather, see it as part of your recovery from anxiety and as an important and supportive force in your healing. Do not be influenced by societal stigma attached to taking psychiatric medications.
- Recognize that medication is not a one-size-fits-all proposition, and that there is a possibility that you may need to try more than one medication before finding the most effective one for you. Your provider can guide you through this process.
- As in any medical appointment, do not feel hesitant or embarrassed to ask questions you may have. Understanding all aspects of your treatment is your right and privilege.

Feeling Safe Again

Anxiety, over all else, convinces us that we are unsafe. The process of anxiety recovery and healing culminates when we once again believe that we are safe from harm and we no longer overprotect or isolate ourselves against perceived danger. When you feel safe again, you have healed. When you no longer wait for disaster to strike, you have healed. When you trust your ability to navigate difficult situations, you have healed. Wherever you are in your healing process, keep moving forward. You are doing great. To those who have just begun their healing journey: without a first step, there can be no further steps. Small progress is still progress. Remind yourself: *I am safe. I am OK. I am safe. I am OK.*

Notes

1 May, R. (1967). *Man's search for meaning.* W.W. Norton & Company.
2 From Zen Mind, Beginner's Mind, by Shunryu Suzuki. Protected under the terms of the International Copyright Union. Reprinted by arrangement with The Permissions Company, Inc., on behalf of Shambhala Publications Inc., Boulder, Colorado, www. shambhala.com.
3 Bandura, A. (1997). *Self-efficacy: The exercise of control.* W. H. Freeman & Company.
4 Forward, S. (2002). *Toxic parents: Overcoming their hurtful legacy and reclaiming your life.* Bantam Books.

4 Tools and Exercises for Coping with IAD

The exercises and examples that follow are intended for use by patients and practitioners as helpful ways to cope with and heal from illness-related anxiety.

Guided Visualization: Safe Space

Visualization is a way to use our imaginations to create cognitive and emotional "safe spaces" that we can access when we are feeling overwhelmed or anxious. The following is an example of a guided visualization.

Find a quiet, soothing space and sit quietly. Gently close your eyes and place both hands on your chest, over your heart. Allow yourself to relax by taking a series of deep breaths, inhaling through your nose and exhaling through your mouth.

When you are ready, bring up an image in your mind of a safe and calming place or scene. It may be a real or an imagined place. Perhaps it is a peaceful clearing in a forest or a comfortable room decorated in a pleasing way. Whatever this place is for you, in it, you are completely and totally safe. Nothing in this place can harm you in any way.

Take note of all the aspects of this place, all the details, even the most minute. Imagine what it might sound like or smell like in this calm and safe place. Take note of the colors in this place, and the feel of the air and the atmosphere. Continuing to take deep breaths from your diaphragm, feel that you are physically in this serene and safe place. Stay here in this safe and secure space for as long as you wish.

Know that you may return to this place anytime you are feeling uneasy, overwhelmed, or worried. This space is yours and yours alone. When you are ready, gently and lovingly open your eyes, stretch, and return your consciousness to the room.

DOI: 10.4324/9781032637921-4

Meditation: Body Scan

A body scan meditation allows you to feel present with your physicality rather than detached from it. When we pay attention to our bodies with loving kindness, we feel whole and safe within them. The following is an example of a body scan meditation.

Take a series of deep breaths, inhaling through your nose and exhaling through your mouth. This meditation can be done sitting up or lying down, whatever is most comfortable for you. However you position yourself, be sure you are comfortable and at ease. Gently close your eyes and focus on your breathing, seeing your breaths as soft ocean waves that go in and out, in and out.

Bring your awareness to the top of your head. Your head houses and protects your brain, which allows you to think, work, and imagine. Stay focused on this part of your body for a moment, paying attention to it. Allow yourself to feel gratitude for the role it plays in your overall health.

When you are ready, shift your attention to your neck and shoulders, noticing how they feel and if there are any points of tightness or tension. Allow those tense parts to relax and let go, all the while continuing to breathe in and out, gentle as calm ocean waves. Your neck and shoulders provide you with mobility and stability. Allow yourself to feel gratitude for the important role they play.

When you feel ready to move on, shift your gentle attention to your chest and the area around your heart. This part of your body pumps and distributes blood and ensures that you receive the oxygen you need. Lovingly allow any tension or tightness in this area to lift. Allow your heart to beat at its own pace, observing it and feeling amazement at its ability to know what to do and how to keep you alive.

Next, move your attention down to your legs, calves, and feet. This part of your body allows you to walk, run, dance, and play. Send gratitude and thankfulness to your legs and feet for the important work they do. Become aware of how they feel and allow them to rest and relax, sending gentle gratitude all the way down to the very ends of your toes.

Now, just allow yourself to be in your body. You don't need to be anywhere else in this moment. Stay here for as long as you wish. Trust your body to keep you alive and safe, all its systems functioning as they should, your heart, brain, lungs, muscles, and bones all doing their unique and important work.

When you are ready and when it feels right for you, slowly open your eyes. Continuing to breathe deeply, come back to the room while still feeling comfortable and at peace within your incredible body. Allow yourself a long stretch, noticing once more all the unique areas of your body and feeling grateful for them.

Meditation: Heart Space/Self-Soothing

Your "heart space" is your chest area, the part of your body that houses your heart and your emotions. By paying gentle attention to it, you are offering yourself soothing and calming. Because this part of your body often responds to and houses stress, anxiety, panic, and worry, it also needs to be reminded at times to be peaceful and still. The following meditation focuses on your heart space.

Sitting upright but not rigid, allow yourself to settle into a comfortable position. When you are ready, gently place both hands over your heart space. Allow your chest and heart to feel warmed and embraced.

Begin taking a series of deep breaths, inhaling through your nose and exhaling through your mouth. Close your eyes and simply sit in this position. You don't need to do anything. Just sit and be, continuing to breathe and paying attention to your breath. As thoughts come, allow them to gently appear and pass, appear and pass. Appear and pass.

Feel the warmth and gentle touch of your hands upon your heart space, offering yourself soothing, healing, and calming. Breathe, in and out, in and out. Remind yourself that you don't need to do anything right now. Just sit. And be.

You may continue to remain in this position for as long as is comfortable for you. When you feel ready, slowly shift your hands away from your heart space, resting them on your legs, and open your eyes. Gently allow yourself to come back to the room and to your conscious awareness.

Exercise: Mantras

Mantras are simple, easy-to-remember and easily accessible statements and affirmations that you can say to yourself when you need them, particularly in times of stress, worry, and overwhelm. The idea is to speak to yourself in a kind, loving, and reassuring way with gentle reminders that you are safe. You can create your own mantras that work for you, asking yourself what you might need to hear in times of worry. For some people, mantras are as simple as statements like "I am OK," or "I am safe," or requests like "may I be safe and free from harm."

Consider what mantras might be helpful to you. Use the space below to list them.

My Mantras

1. I am safe.

2.

3.

4.

5.

CBT Exercise: Challenging Anxious Assumptions

It is impossible not to have thoughts. You experience thousands of unique thoughts during the course of a day, most with a duration of less than five seconds. It is only natural that some of those thoughts will have an anxious tone. When we experience anxious or uncomfortable thoughts, it can be easy to simply believe them and draw anxiety-driven assumptions and conclusions. Cognitive behavioral therapy teaches us to examine our anxious thoughts and their resulting assumptions and conclusions instead of accepting them as factual. Use this chart as a framework for challenging your anxiety-based assumptions.

Situation	Thought	Assumption	Challenge to Assumption
Example: I have a physical check-up tomorrow.	The doctor may find something wrong with me.	A doctor's office is a place where you find out bad news.	A physical check-up is a way for me to stay on top of my health.

CBT Exercise: Challenging Automatic Thoughts

Automatic thoughts are thoughts that arise reflexively in direct response to a situation or stimulus. For example, an anxious person may hear a sound in the night and automatically assume that the house is being broken into. The problem with automatic thoughts is that they take a knee-jerk form, leaving us no room for closer inspection as to their accuracy.

Use this chart below as a framework to challenge your automatic thoughts.

Event	Automatic Thought	Challenge to Automatic Thought	New Thought
Example: I experience chest pain.	"I am having a heart attack."	"I have no other symptoms; it might not be a heart attack."	"I am uncomfortable right now, but I am not in danger."

CBT Exercise: Feelings and Physiology

Tracking the effects of anxiety, stress, and worry on your body can be helpful in gaining an understanding of your unique physical responses and where your feelings "live" inside your body. Use the chart below to track your physiological response to the "big three" emotions of fear, anger, and sadness.

Fear/Anxiety	*Anger*	*Sadness*
Example: My chest/heart	My head	My muscles

CBT Exercise: Emotion and Behavioral Response

In an anxious state, we tend to have an immediate behavioral response to our emotions. Learning to pause and create cognitive "space" between our feelings related to an event or situation and our behavioral responses is important in reducing our tendency to respond without thinking rationally and calmly.

Example:

Anxiety-Based Response

Event (something happens):
I experience chest tightness.

Emotion (I feel something):
I feel frightened.

Behavioral Response (I do something):
I go to the emergency room.

Rational Response

Event:
I experience chest tightness.

Emotion:
I feel frightened.

Behavioral Response:
I don't need to do anything in this moment. I can check in with myself in a little while and see how I am feeling then.

Based on the example above, use this template as a framework to sketch out a rational response to an event or situation:

Event:

Emotion:

Behavioral Response:

CBT Exercise: Probability Overestimations

Anxiety often overestimates likelihoods and turns possibilities into probabilities. Being aware of our tendency to overestimate the probability of certain outcomes is a way to challenge anxious thinking. Use the chart below to track your feared outcomes related to situations and to remind yourself that in many cases, the outcome you fear is not probable.

Situation	Feared Outcome	Possibility or Probability
Example: I feel groin pain.	I have testicular cancer	There is a *possibility* of this, but the *probability* is much lower.

DBT Exercise: "Wise Mind"[1]

Dialectical behavioral therapy teaches us to find a healthy overlap between our emotional and our rational minds. This midpoint, or "Wise Mind," is a place where we are attuned to "what is" and where we operate from a perspective of self-trust and intuition rather than fear and anxiety.

Use the chart below to help find the "wise point" that intersects your emotional and rational thoughts.

Rational Thought	Emotional Thought	Wise Thought
"It is difficult to swallow."	"I can't breathe/I am going to die."	This is frightening, but I have had a sore throat recently and it may just be irritation. I can wait a few days and see if it resolves. I can also take other measures to see if it feels better before taking any drastic action.

Narrative Therapy Exercise: Write a Letter to Your Anxiety

The act of putting words around our uncomfortable emotions can have a healing quality. The more we allow unpleasant feelings to be unspoken, the more they fester and take up emotional space within us. Writing to our problem is a way to address it directly and, therefore, feel that we have some power over it and that it does not control us.

The following letter addresses anxiety in a gentle, rather than aggressive or hostile, tone that allows for an understanding of what anxiety does and how the writer plans to manage it. In a way, the exercise of writing it down, in a way, makes it real.

Dear Anxiety,

I've gotten to know you well over the past few years. I know where you live in my body, and I know, too, that when you come around you are trying to keep me safe. But sometimes you try too hard and it makes me feel afraid. I've decided that when you come, I am going to gently turn your volume down. This doesn't mean I will never listen to you but, rather, that I will not let you overwhelm me. I would like to thank you for the times when you've reminded me to be mindful and cautious. I know you have good intentions and that you want me to be safe. But I would like to use you in a way that is helpful to me.

Sincerely,

Consider what a letter written to your anxiety or panic might sound like. Use the space below to write it.

Letter to My Anxiety
Dear Anxiety,
Sincerely,

Exercise: Soothing Activities

Having a bank of soothing activities that we can access when we are feeling overly anxious is helpful in redirecting our anxious energy toward healthier endeavors. Your list should include even the simplest activities, as they can be just as soothing and healthily distracting as more complex activities.

Go for a short walk.
Sit with, play with, or pet your dog or cat.
Get some fresh air.
Listen to calming music.
Work on a crossword puzzle, sudoku, word search, or other game or puzzle.
Do a short, simple meditation.
Take a warm shower or a relaxing bath.

Consider what other soothing activities you might add to your list. Use the space below to compile them.

My Soothing Activities
1. Go for a short walk.
2.
3.
4.
5.

Mindfulness Exercise: Coping Statements

Coping statements are short sentences that we can utilize to remind ourselves that we are safe when we are experiencing heightened anxiety, panic, or worry. These statements can take any form that you find helpful. They may sound like the following:

"I have felt this way before and I have been OK."
"I feel uncomfortable right now, but this feeling is temporary."
"In this moment, I am safe."
"I can do what I need to relax in this moment."
"It is OK for me to rest right now."
"All feelings pass. No feeling is permanent."
"My feelings are uncomfortable right now, but I can accept them."
"Anxious thoughts are not predictions or facts."

Consider what your own coping statements might sound like. Use the space below to list them.

My Coping Statements
1. My feelings are uncomfortable right now, but I can accept them.
2.
3.
4.
5.

Exercise: Knowing My Personal Anxiety Centers

Every individual's body stores stress and anxiety differently. Therefore, it is important to understand your body's unique way of reacting to fear and anxiety. Understanding where anxiety is housed in your body can help you care for yourself when you are experiencing intense physical symptoms. Use the diagram below to mark the places in your body where you typically experience stress responses so that you can accurately interpret the symptoms when they occur (see Figure 4.1).

MY ANXIETY CENTERS

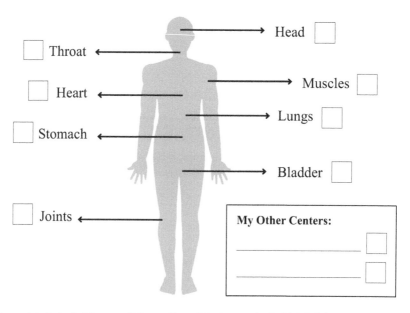

Figure 4.1 A shaded image of the outline of the human body highlighting areas where readers can mark off checkboxes to show places where their bodies respond to anxiety.

Exercise: Triggers Action Plan

Understanding what triggers us is important in cultivating an ability to prepare for triggers and to respond to them in a healthy, soothing way. Keeping a working list of the situations or events that cause you to have an emotional response and considering what you need in those moments can help you to feel that you have a plan to care for yourself when you are feeling triggered. Use the chart below to keep track of your triggers, the emotions they bring up, and your plan for coping.

Trigger	*Emotion*	*Action Plan*
Example: Chest pain	Fear/Panic	Do my "Safe Space" Visualization

Note

1 Linehan, M. M., & Linehan, M. (2015). *DBT skills training manual*. The Guilford Press. Manning, James & Nicola Ridgeway. *CBT Worksheets*. Suffolk, Great Britain, West Suffolk CBT Service, LTD., 2016.

Bibliography

Almalki, M., Al-Tawayjri, I., Al-Anazi, A., Mahmoud, S., & Al-Mohrej, A. (2016). A recommendation for the management of illness anxiety disorder patients abusing the health care system. *Case Reports in Psychiatry, 2016,* 1–3. https://doi.org/10.1155/2016/6073598

American Psychiatric Association. (2022). *Diagnostic and statistical manual of mental disorders* (5th ed., text rev.). American Psychiatric Association.

Bandura, A. (1997). *Self-efficacy: The exercise of control.* W. H. Freeman & Company.

Beck, A. T. (1991). *Cognitive therapy and the emotional disorders.* Penguin Books.

Caron, C. (2022, October 29). Teens turn to TikTok in search of a mental health diagnosis. *New York Times.* www.nytimes.com/2022/10/29/well/mind/tiktok-mental-illness-diagnosis.html

Casanova-Perez, R., Apodaca, C., Bascom, E., Mohanraj, D., Lane, C., Vidyarthi, D., Beneteau, E., Sabin, J., Pratt, W., Weibel, N., & Hartzler, A. L. (2022a, February 21). Broken down by bias: Healthcare biases experienced by BIPOC and LGBTQ+ patients. *AMIA Annual Symposium Proceedings, 2021,* 275–84.

Casanova-Perez, R., Apodaca, C., Bascom, E., Mohanraj, D., Lane, C., Vidyarthi, D., Beneteau, E., Sabin, J., Pratt, W., Weibel, N., & Hartzler, A. L. (2022b, February 21). Broken down by bias: Healthcare biases experienced by BIPOC and LGBTQ+ patients. *AMIA Annual Symposium Proceedings.* AMIA Symposium. Retrieved April 2, 2023, from www.ncbi.nlm.nih.gov/pmc/articles/PMC8861755/

Ellis, A., & Ellis, D. (2019). *Rational emotive behavioral therapy.* American Psychological Association.

Forward, S. (2002). *Toxic parents: Overcoming their hurtful legacy and reclaiming your life.* Bantam Books.

Freud, S. (1963). *General psychological theory.* Collier Bks.

Herman, J. L. (2015). *Trauma and recovery.* Pandora.

Linehan, M. M., & Linehan, M. (2015). *DBT skills training manual.* The Guilford Press.

Manning, James & Nicola Ridgeway. *CBT Worksheets.* Suffolk, Great Britain, West Suffolk CBT Service, LTD., 2016.

May, R. (1967). *Man's search for meaning.* W.W. Norton & Company.

National Center for Health Statistics. (2022, December 8). *Mortality in the United States, 2021.* Centers for Disease Control and Prevention. www.cdc.gov/nchs/products/databriefs/db456.htm#section_4

National Institute for Occupational Safety and Health. (2022, May 11). *Health worker mental health*. Centers for Disease Control and Prevention. www.cdc.gov/niosh/newsroom/feature/health-worker-mental-health.html

Ravan, J. R., Chatterjee, S., Singh, P., Maikap, D., & Padhan, P. (2021, June 30). Autoimmune rheumatic diseases masquerading as psychiatric disorders: A case series. *Mediterranean Journal of Rheumatology*, *32*(2), 164–67. https://doi.org/10.31138/mjr.32.2.164

Skinner, M. (2014). Environmental stress and epigenetic transgenerational inheritance. *BMC Medicine*, *12*(153). https://doi.org/10.1186/s12916-014-0153-y

Suzuki, S. (1987). *Zen mind, beginner's mind*. Shambhala Publications.

White, M., & Epston, D. (1990). *Narrative means to therapeutic ends*. W.W. Norton & Company.

Wolynn, M. (2022). *It didn't start with you: How inherited family trauma shapes who we are and how to end the cycle*. Vermilion.

Index

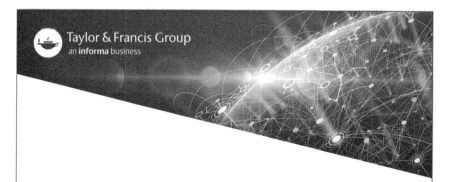